FOOD SOLUTIONS
Premenstrual Syndrome

FOOD SOLUTIONS
Premenstrual Syndrome

Recipes and Advice to Control Symptons

Patsy Westcott

hamlyn

Safety note

This book should not be considered a replacement for professional medical treament. A doctor should be consulted on all matters relating to health; particularly in respect of any symptoms which may require diagnosis or medical attention. While the advice and information in this book are believed to be accurate, neither the author nor the publisher can accept any legal responsibility for any injury or illness sustained while following the treatments and diet plan.

Natural Health Advisory Service
PO Box 268
Lewes
East Sussex
BN7 1QN

Website: http://www.wnas.org.uk
Telephone: 01273 487366

First published in Great Britain in 2002 by
Hamlyn, a division of Octopus Publishing Group Ltd
2–4 Heron Quays, London E14 4JP

This revised edition published 2004

Copyright © Octopus Publishing Group Ltd 2002, 2004

ISBN 0 600 61056 X

A CIP catalogue record for this book is available from the British Library

Printed and bound in the United Kingdom by MacKays of Chatham

10 9 8 7 6 5 4 3 2 1

Contents

Introduction

It was the Greek father of medicine, Hippocrates, who in ancient times first described 'the shivering, lassitude and heaviness of head that denotes the onset of menstruation'. But although premenstrual syndrome (PMS), or premenstrual tension (PMT) as it used to be called, has been recognized for thousands of years, it was by no means the scourge it is today. The changes in women's lives that came about in the 20th century mean that many women today lead very different lives to previous generations. In our grandmothers' day, women started their periods later, had more pregnancies and died younger – all of which meant fewer menstrual cycles and less PMS.

Today one in three women are estimated to endure the monthly misery of PMS. Symptoms commonly include bloating, breast tenderness, fatigue, headaches, weight gain, irritability and fluctuations in mood. One in twenty suffer an extreme and disabling form of PMS known as PDD (premenstrual dysphoric disorder) which causes more severe depression, anxiety and mood swings.

The good news is that doctors and scientists are at last beginning to solve the riddle of PMS. Research that has been carried out over the past few years has focused more and more on the links between the brain and the body rather than simply on the ups and downs of the female sex hormones, oestrogen and progesterone.

Many doctors now argue that women with PMS are in fact probably oversensitive, physically and mentally, to normal fluctuations in their hormones. With this realization, it is becoming increasingly apparent that every woman has the potential to develop PMS. This new understanding is leading to some promising new treatments and also to a greater awareness of things women can do for themselves to successfully raise their PMS threshold.

This book is designed to help you do just that by helping you understand more about the potential causes of PMS and by providing you with ideas to help you manage your symptoms more effectively.

Chapter 1 describes what happens in the menstrual cycle and explains the role of various hormones that are involved in this finely orchestrated process.

Chapter 2 outlines some of the predominant symptoms of PMS and looks at some of the theories relating to its causes. It also identifies different types and patterns of PMS and gives advice on when to see the doctor and how to get the most out of a consultation.

Chapter 3 is all about how to help yourself with PMS. It explains how keeping a menstrual calendar can enable you to find out if you really have PMS. It also provides a wealth of easy-to-follow advice and practical tips on ways to adjust your lifestyle and either banish the symptoms of PMS, or minimize their effects.

Chapter 4 outlines some of the many treatments that are available, both over the counter in pharmacies and health food shops, and on prescription from the doctor. It includes vitamins and minerals and some of the herbal treatments that are becoming increasingly popular. There's also information on other treatment approaches, such as cognitive therapy, light therapy and surgery.

In Chapter 5 you will find a rundown of complementary treatments that some women have found helpful in controlling their symptoms. Some complementary therapies are now becoming the subject of mainstream clinical research and in the next few years look set to offer a natural but effective solution to some of the symptoms of PMS.

One the most important things you can do if you suffer PMS is to pay attention to what you eat. Nutrient deficiencies can play a significant part in lowering the threshold of PMS and taking steps to make sure you eat a healthy, nutritious diet can do a great deal to free you from symptoms. Chapter 6 gathers together all that has been discovered about the various dietary and nutritional factors that may play a part in PMS, and gives practical advice on how to moderate your eating and drinking habits to banish or minimize symptoms.

Finally, Chapter 7 contains a wide range of delicious recipes designed to help you put all these ideas into practice.

1 The menstrual cycle

Understanding the menstrual cycle is the first piece in putting together the jigsaw of premenstrual syndrome (PMS). The average age of girls having their first period today is 12 years, and the average age of women at the onset of the menopause is 51. This, coupled with the availability of contraception which has led to fewer pregnancies, means that the average woman nowadays will have some 470 menstrual cycles during the course of her reproductive life. It's not surprising, therefore, that there is such a plague of PMS.

An understanding of how your body works and what can go wrong will help you gain control over your symptoms. This chapter provides an overview of the menstrual cycle, how it works and how it might contribute to your PMS. It describes in detail what happens each month as your body prepares itself for a possible pregnancy. It also outlines the role played by the endocrine – or glandular – system in this process, and the effects it can have on the rest of your body.

That time of the month

The word menstruation, from which the term 'menstrual cycle' derives, comes from the Latin word *mensis*, meaning month. The menstrual cycle is defined as the time span from the first day of one menstrual period to the first day of the next one.

Every month from puberty until the menopause – unless suppressed, for example by pregnancy, breastfeeding or the contraceptive pill – this intricate and finely tuned pattern of activity prepares your body to nourish a new life, by lining the womb ready to accept a fertilized egg. If an egg is not fertilized that month, the lining of the womb, or uterus, falls away in the form of a period or menstruation.

Although, for convenience sake, a normal menstrual cycle is usually calculated as 28 days, in fact a 28-day cycle is relatively rare and many women have shorter or longer cycles – anything from 24–40 days.

During each cycle, the reproductive organs undergo a series of changes under the influence of hormones that cause a follicle, a sac containing an egg or ovum, to mature in the ovary. At ovulation, the egg is released from the follicle into the abdominal cavity from where it finds its way into the Fallopian tubes and travels down to the uterus.

If fertilization does not occur, the egg, together with the lining of the womb (the endometrium) is shed in the menstrual flow, allowing a new lining to grow, ready to nurture another potential pregnancy. Menstruation lasts on average for four to five days, but again the length of time varies greatly from woman to woman and bleeding can last anything from three to ten days.

Phases of the menstrual cycle

The menstrual cycle has three different phases.

The menstrual phase or menstruation

This accounts for day one to about day five of your cycle. During this phase the endometrium, or lining of the womb, is shed. The tissue and blood pass out through your vagina as a period. By the fifth day, the growing ovarian follicles are starting to produce more oestrogen.

The follicular or proliferative phase

This is days 6–14 of your menstrual cycle, when the follicle or egg sac develops. During this phase the endometrium regrows under the influence of rising levels of oestrogen. The womb lining becomes thick, velvety and rich in blood vessels. Rising oestrogen levels also cause the cervical mucus to become thin and stretchy like egg white, so that sperm can easily pass through into the uterus. Ovulation marks the end of the follicular phase. It takes place 14 days before the onset of a period, so in a 28-day cycle, ovulation will happen around day 14. In a 24-day cycle, ovulation will take place on or around day 11, while in a 40-day cycle ovulation will occur around day 26.

The luteal or secretory phase

This is days 15-28 of the menstrual cycle. It is during this phase that PMS symptoms develop, although the precise trigger is not fully understood. During the secretory phase, rising progesterone levels increase the blood supply to the uterus, creating a blood- and nutrient-rich environment within the uterus in preparation for a potential embryo. Rising progesterone levels cause the cervical mucus to become thick and viscous, forming a plug at the entrance to the uterus which prevents sperm from entering.

Towards the end of this phase, if fertilization has not taken place, progesterone levels then fall. This deprives the endometrium of oxygen and nutrients and causes the cells to die, paving the way for the endometrium to be sloughed off during menstruation.

Hormones and the menstrual cycle

The menstrual cycle is governed by the action of hormones secreted by the glands of the body's endocrine, or hormonal, system. From the moment we are conceived until the day we die, our bodies are under the influence of a cocktail of hormones produced by our glands. The ovaries have two roles in the body: they are organs of the reproductive system, storing and producing eggs, and they are also glands of the endocrine system, producing the female sex hormones, which are oestrogen and progesterone.

Hormones are chemical messengers that travel around in the bloodstream to act on cells and tissues around the body. Each hormone is responsible for acting on one specific type of tissue only.

In order to ensure that hormones don't latch on to any cell at random, the cells have special receptors on their surfaces or inside, onto which the correct hormones can lock rather like a key fitting into a keyhole. This means hormones can be transported in the bloodstream to their destination without going astray.

The glands of the endocrine system all work together to make sure that our bodies stay in a constant state of balance or homeostasis. This is made possible by a series of feedback mechanisms that slow or stop the activity of a particular gland once enough of a hormone has been produced, and turn it on again when more is needed, a bit like a central-heating thermostat. This system is so delicately balanced that, if anything happens to disturb it, the repercussions can be felt throughout the whole body. One reason why premenstrual syndrome can have such far reaching consequences throughout the body is because of this interaction between the different parts of the endocrine system.

The hypothalamus, the pituitary and the ovaries

The menstrual cycle itself is under the control of a feedback loop, which operates between the hypothalamus (the part of the brain that controls hormone production), the pituitary gland (the body's master gland) and the ovaries.

The hypothalamus is a region of the brain, about the size of a cherry, with nerve connections to most other parts of the nervous system. It controls the autonomic nervous system (which controls automatic functions beyond our conscious control, such as breathing and heart rate) and coordinates the function of the nervous and endocrine systems.

The pituitary is pea-sized structure at the base of the brain, referred to as the body's master gland because it is the most important in the endocrine system. It regulates and controls the activities of all the other endocrine glands and many other body processes. Among the many hormones it secretes are the gonadotrophins, the follicle-stimulating hormone (FSH) and luteinizing hormone (LH), which stimulate the ovaries to produce oestrogen and progesterone.

The hypothalamus is connected to the pituitary by a short stalk of nerve fibres. Through direct nerve connections and the secretion of chemicals called hormone-releasing factors, the hypothalamus controls hormonal secretions from the pituitary. In this way, indirectly via the pituitary, the hypothalamus controls many of the glands of the endocrine system, including the ovaries.

The connections between the hypothalamus, the pituitary and the ovaries are currently the subject of a great deal of scientific investigation which is revealing some intriguing clues as to the causes of PMS. Some of the new theories emerging are explored in the next chapter.

Raging hormones

On the first day of your menstrual cycle, the hypothalamus produces a hormone called GnRH (Gonadotrophin-releasing hormone). This triggers the pituitary to produce a chemical messenger called follicle-stimulating hormone (FSH) and a luteinizing hormone (LH). FSH travels in the bloodstream to the ovaries where it stimulates the follicles to develop. It also triggers the secretion of oestrogen by the ovaries.

Rising levels of oestrogen in the blood in turn trigger a lowering of FSH in a negative feedback loop, just enough to allow one follicle and its egg to ripen. At the same time, oestrogen causes the endometrium (womb lining) to become juicy and thick in preparation for receiving a fertilized egg. Oestrogen also stimulates the build-up of body proteins, which leads to the body retaining more fluid.

As oestrogen levels begin to peak around mid-cycle, they trigger a sudden surge of another hormone, luteinizing hormone (LH), from the pituitary. This stimulates the ripe egg to burst from its follicle, a process known as ovulation, about 36 hours later.

LH now goes into action to cause the development of the corpus luteum in the empty follicle. Its job is further to prepare the body for a pregnancy. The corpus luteum makes and releases its own hormone, progesterone, which sensitizes the tissue of the breasts, uterine lining and vaginal walls. Levels of progesterone rise and peak around day 21.

If the egg is not fertilized, the corpus luteum shrinks, the egg disintegrates and progesterone levels plummet. This in turn causes the blood vessels in the endometrium to break and the uterus fills with blood and tissue. The uterine walls contract to expel this in the form of a period.

The decline in progesterone and oestrogen levels stops the blockade of FSH and LH, and the whole cycle starts anew.

The endocrine system

The endocrine system consists of hormone-producing glands. Many of these are regulated by stimulating hormones produced by the pituitary gland. The pituitary is in turn influenced by releasing hormones secreted by the hypothalamus, situated at the base of the brain. The hypothalamus-pituitary-thyroid axis is particularly important in PMS.

Hypothalamus

Hypothalamic hormones stimulate the pituitary. The hypothalamus helps control appetite, weight control, sleep, sexual desire, mood and emotion.

Pineal gland

This responds to dark and light and may be linked to sexual development.

Pituitary gland

This secretes hormones that stimulate the adrenal glands, the thyroid, pigment-producing skin cells and the ovaries or testes. It also secretes the growth hormone, antidiuretic hormone, prolactin and oxytocin, which partly causes the uterus to contract in childbirth and during periods.

Parathyroid gland

This regulates calcium concentration in the blood.

Thyroid gland

This helps stimulate metabolism, body temperature and bone growth. Its activity is controlled by stimulating hormones produced by the pituitary.

Thymus gland

This plays a vital part in immunity and resistance of infection.

Ovaries

These produce oestrogen and progesterone, which influence virtually every aspect of female physiology including skin, hair, body composition, bone density and reproductive function. They are governed by gonadotrophic hormones produced by the pituitary.

Adrenal cortex

Adrenal cortical-stimulating hormone (ACTH), produced by the pituitary, causes the adrenal glands to produce hydrocortisone, which effects the metabolism. They also produce androgens (male sex hormones) and aldosterone, which regulate blood pressure and the body's salt balance.

Pancreas

The pancreas secretes insulin and glucagon, which control energy in the body.

2 Understanding premenstrual syndrome

Practically every woman of reproductive age experiences some changes in physical and mental wellbeing before a period. However, not all women experience them to the extent that they interfere with their daily lives. Of those that do, most experience only mild to moderate disruption. But, for an unlucky few, PMS can be so disabling that their whole lives revolve around 'that time of the month'. The precise causes of PMS have yet to be fully unravelled, but in the past few years scientists have begun to uncover a number of intriguing clues.

This chapter looks at what PMS is, giving a rundown of some of the most commonly reported symptoms and some of the different types of PMS. It also details some theories of what causes PMS and outlines some discoveries that are leading to a better understanding of PMS and how it may be treated.

Finally, it offers practical information and tips on when you should see the doctor and how the doctor might make a diagnosis. This can help to put you on the path to a PMS-free life, or at the very least help you to reduce the intensity of your symptoms.

What is premenstrual syndrome?

Virtually all women notice some physical and mental alterations in the run-up to their period. What defines PMS is that these changes are sufficiently pronounced to have an impact on your daily life.

PMS has been known since ancient times, but it was only in 1931 that it was given a name by an American neurologist. Since that time, 150 physical and mental symptoms have been identified and between 80 and 300 different treatments developed. In many ways PMS is a paradox: every woman afflicted with it can describe its effects and yet doctors still disagree on how to define it, and its underlying causes remain a mystery.

The symptoms

The symptoms are not unique to PMS. In fact many of them can be signs of other disorders, such as depression and thyroid problems. Nor are they confined to women. Men, too, can experience many of the individual symptoms of PMS, such as irritability, anger and headaches. Just to confuse matters further, the symptoms of PMS can vary both from cycle to cycle and from woman to woman. This has led doctors to surmise that different underlying mechanisms may be at work in different women.

The defining feature of PMS is its timing. Symptoms occur every month, anything from 2–14 days before the start of the menstrual cycle. For most women the symptoms stop at the onset of menstruation and disappear altogether during the early phase of the menstrual cycle.

The symptoms of PMS can be broadly divided into physical changes, such as bloating and breast tenderness; alterations in mood, such as depression, mood swings and irritability; and cognitive changes, that is changes in concentration, memory and attention. You will find the most common ones summarized below.

Mood changes

❑ Altered interest in sex
❑ Anger and aggression
❑ Anxiety
❑ Depression
❑ Edginess
❑ Exacerbation of existing mental health problems, such as depression
❑ Fatigue and tiredness
❑ Food cravings
❑ Irritability
❑ Mood swings
❑ Tearfulness

Cognitive changes

❑ Accident proneness
❑ Confusion
❑ Difficulty sticking to a task

- ❏ Forgetfulness
- ❏ Lack of coordination

Physical changes

- ❏ Acne and rashes
- ❏ Abdominal pain or cramping
- ❏ Appetite changes
- ❏ Backache and other aches and pains
- ❏ Bloating
- ❏ Breast tenderness
- ❏ Changes in bowel habits
- ❏ Changes in energy level
- ❏ Exacerbation of existing physical complaints
- ❏ Headaches
- ❏ Migraines
- ❏ Muscle or joint stiffness
- ❏ Puffiness of face, abdomen, ankles, fingers
- ❏ Sleep disturbances
- ❏ Weight gain

How serious is PMS?

Because the symptoms of PMS disappear at menstruation without treatment, and are not progressive or life-threatening, doctors don't classify PMS as a serious illness. If your life is turned upside down by bloating, mood swings, headaches and other depressing and debilitating symptoms for a week or so of every month, it can be distressing to be told that your suffering is not serious.

This is not to say that it shouldn't be taken seriously, however. If PMS is affecting your quality of life, it's a good idea to get it properly diagnosed by a doctor, both to rule out other medically treatable conditions, and to try and find a way to manage it more effectively.

How common is PMS?

Although this is an apparently simple question, the incidence of PMS is frustratingly hard to pin down. A study of some of the books and articles on PMS written for doctors and patients throws up the following conflicting statements:

- ❑ 'At least 60 per cent of all women suffer from PMS'
- ❑ 'As many as eight out of ten women have physical and emotional symptoms of premenstrual syndrome, or PMS'
- ❑ 'PMS...affects about 5 per cent of women'
- ❑ 'PMS...affects up to 40 per cent of women of child bearing age'
- ❑ 'From 10–90 per cent of women have PMS at some time during their menstruating years'
- ❑ '50–80 per cent of menstruating women report having some degree of premenstrual symptoms'
- ❑ '...as many as 85 per cent of menstruating women experience one or more of the symptoms of PMS'

Practically the only thing these experts agree on is that they disagree! This disparity is partly to do with the wide range of symptoms associated with PMS, and partly to do with the difficulties in defining it. Suffice to say that PMS is extremely common and that if you have it you are not alone.

Who gets PMS?

PMS can affect any woman of reproductive age and symptoms can start anytime from puberty to the menopause. Symptoms are relieved during pregnancy and after the menopause, although some women experience similar symptoms if they have hormone replacement therapy (HRT) of the type in which both oestrogen and progestogen are given.

Symptoms often start in the twenties and become particularly troublesome in the early to mid-thirties. Many women report that symptoms are triggered or worsened by hormonal changes in the body, for example coming off the pill, pregnancy, termination, hysterectomy and other kinds of pelvic surgery. Some women experience fewer symptoms as they approach the menopause. However, as with so many other aspects of PMS, this is by no means a general rule and some find that their symptoms worsen.

What's in a name? PMT, PMS and PDD

PMS didn't become a major popular concern until the 1960s and 1970s with the growth of feminism. For a long while it was generally referred to as premenstrual tension or PMT, but in the 1980s the term premenstrual syndrome (PMS) became widespread, reflecting the fact that the condition can be both physical and mental. A syndrome is a collection of symptoms that appear together forming a pattern typical of a condition.

In more recent years, the term premenstrual dysphoric disorder (PMDD or PDD) has appeared. The term dysphoria means lowered mood (the opposite of euphoria) and the symptoms of PDD are primarily, though not entirely, related to mood. They include:

❑ Anger or irritability

❑ Anxiety and tension

❑ Changes in appetite – either wanting to eat more or less

- ❑ Depression
- ❑ Difficulty concentrating
- ❑ Loss of interest in usual activities such as sex
- ❑ Fatigue
- ❑ Mood swings
- ❑ Sleep disturbances
- ❑ Physical symptoms that may include breast pain, bloating and headaches.

There is still debate among doctors about whether PDD is the same as PMS, a separate mood disorder tied to the menstrual cycle or a particularly debilitating form of PMS.

Current thinking seems to be that approximately three to five per cent of women suffer PDD, which mainly involves disturbances in mood. Like PMS, symptoms occur during the last week or so of the menstrual cycle and remit during the early part of the cycle.

A diagnosis of PDD requires at least one marked mood change – such as depression, hopelessness, anxiety, tension, anger or irritability – and symptoms must be severe enough to seriously disrupt daily life.

Studies have shown that women with PDD face a higher risk of developing clinical depression at some time in their lives. Furthermore, between three and six out of ten women suffering depression experience an exacerbation of symptoms before a period. Having said that, PDD and clinical depression are two separate conditions.

What causes PMS?

The exact causes of premenstrual syndrome have yet to be identified, and while some experts attribute the symptoms of

PMS OR PDD?

Tick the circles which you feel describe your symptoms:

○ Your symptoms mainly affect your mood
○ You experience five or more of the following symptoms:

Mood swings

Depression

Irritability

Lack of interest in your usual activities

Difficulty concentrating

Lack of energy

Marked change in appetite

Difficulty sleeping or sleeping a lot

Feeling overwhelmed

Bloating and breast tenderness

Tension.

○ Your symptoms interfere with your work.
○ Your symptoms interfere with your social life.
○ Your symptoms interfere with domestic activities.
○ Your symptoms affect your relationships with family and friends.
○ Your symptoms occur only in the week or two before your period.
○ You experience symptoms most cycles.
○ You have experienced symptoms over at least two consecutive cycles.
○ Symptoms stop once you get your period.

If you've ticked every circle, you may have PDD as well as, or rather than, PMS. Talk to your doctor.

PMS to a hormonal imbalance in the body, others argue that an imbalance in brain chemicals during the menstrual cycle is more likely to cause PMS.

Hormonal links

The timing of PMS symptoms seems to point strongly to a hormonal connection. Until the last decade or so, many doctors believed that PMS was linked to a straighforward hormonal imbalance – for example a shortage of progesterone or oestrogen. Unfortunately, research failed to find a clear-cut hormonal cause and studies of blood levels show that there are no differences between women with and without PMS. In the past few years, this theory has given way to a clearer understanding of how hormones may be involved.

The brain-body connection

One of the most popular current hypotheses is that the origins of PMS may lie not in the reproductive system at all but in the brain. According to this theory, if you have PMS your brain circuitry may be wired in such a way as to render you hypersensitive to normal fluctuations in your own hormones.

This makes a lot of sense in the light of the fact that most women with PMS are otherwise perfectly healthy. Researchers investigating the chemicals in the brain known as neurotransmitters and neuropeptides, which transmit messages from one nerve cell to another, have found that these chemicals behave differently in women with PMS. They surmise that in women who are sensitive, cyclical changes in levels of progesterone and oestrogen alter the behaviour of these brain chemicals, leading to the symptoms of PMS.

Of course the million-dollar question is why and, unfortunately, the answer is that we still don't know, although there are some clues. However, the recognition of it has paved the way for new treatments for PMS based on correcting imbalances of brain chemicals rather than simply tackling individual symptoms.

The serotonin factor

One of the most important of these brain chemicals is serotonin (or 5-HT), sometimes known as the happiness hormone because of its role in controlling mood. Low serotonin levels are linked to cravings for starchy foods, sleep disorders, depression and mood swings – all symptoms familiar to sufferers of PMS.

Over the past few years, the recognition of the importance of serotonin in controlling mood has led to the development of a class of drugs known as SSRIs (selective serotonin reuptake inhibitors) which act to raise serotonin levels. The most well-known of these is Prozac.

Researchers have found that in women with severe PMS or PDD there is a disturbance in the way serotonin functions during the second phase of their menstrual cycle. In these women, SSRIs can be an extremely effective treatment for reducing emotional symptoms.

However, as with so much else to do with PMS, no one rule applies to every woman.

Other hormones and brain chemicals

Researchers are also beginning to look at other hormones and brain chemicals that may behave in a faulty way.

One of these is a pituitary hormone called prolactin, sometimes known as the mothering hormone for its role in the development of breast tissue and the production of milk during breastfeeding. Prolactin operates in a feedback loop with progesterone, one of the two key female hormones.

Other suspects include a group of neurotransmitters called catecholamines. These include compounds such as noradrenalin, a brain chemical involved in the stress response. High levels of noradrenalin in the brain cause a feeling of elation and low levels cause depression.

Another is dopamine, which affects brain processes that control movement, our emotional response and the ability to experience pleasure or pain.

Another suggestion is that falling levels of progesterone by-products in the blood act on the receptor for another neurotransmitter called gamma-aminobutyric acid or GABA. This blocks the action of nerve cells in certain parts of the brain, causing anxiety, panic attacks and aggression.

Quite how these different chemicals all interact has yet to be fully discovered, however.

The hypothalamic-pituitary-thyroid axis

As we saw in the last chapter, all the body's glands work together in harmony, and if there is an imbalance in one, then it can have knock-on effects on one of the others. Some experts believe that a malfunction of a specific cluster of glands which work together – the hypothalamus, the pituitary and the thyroid gland, found in the neck – may play a part in triggering PMS. The hypothalamus responds to neurotransmitters and may be the link between the ovaries and the brain. As more research is done, the connections between all these factors are likely to become clearer and throw new light on the causes of premenstrual syndrome.

Nutrient shortages

Shortages of nutrients – in particular calcium, magnesium, zinc, B vitamins, and essential fatty acids – have been linked to PMS. Research has found, for example, that over half of PMS sufferers have low levels of magnesium, a mineral closely involved in the action of the brain circuitry.

Other studies have looked at the effect of a shortage of essential fatty acids, which can cause an imbalance of prostaglandins (hormone-like substances that affect many bodily functions).

The nutritional status of women is often not as good as it should be because of aspects of modern life, such as the consumption of processed foods, environmental pollution, smoking and the pill. According to this research, nutrient levels can be further compromised by pregnancy and breastfeeding, leading to nutrient shortages. This may be why PMS often becomes apparent for the first time, or gets worse, after pregnancy or coming off the pill. You will find more details about the role of nutrients in Chapters 4 and 6.

Trigger factors

While the causes of PMS remain baffling, there do seem to be some common triggers – although these don't apply to every woman. It could well be that the condition is triggered by different factors in different women. The following events can often spark off or worsen existing symptoms:

- ❑ The start of menstruation at puberty.
- ❑ The perimenopause (the years approaching your last period).
- ❑ Coming off the contraceptive pill.
- ❑ Giving birth, miscarriage or a termination.
- ❑ Postnatal depression.
- ❑ A spell of no periods (amenorrhoea).
- ❑ A hysterectomy, with or without removal of the ovaries.
- ❑ Certain types of pelvic surgery, especially tubal ligation (an operation rarely performed today in which the Fallopian tubes were tied off).
- ❑ A run of minor illnesses that have left you run down.
- ❑ Major physical or emotional trauma.

Life events and stress

Life events, both negative ones like losing your job, financial difficulties, divorce and bereavement, and happy ones like the birth of a baby, getting a pay rise or getting married, have all been linked to PMS. Researchers have found that chronic stress – the constant everyday ups and downs of life, like getting stuck in a traffic jam, an argument with your partner or struggling financially – are more likely to trigger symptoms than major life events. It is 'the drips rather than the floods' that do us in, as one US psychologist has put it.

Stress may increase the risk of developing PMS in a couple of ways. Firstly, it raises levels of cortisol, one of the stress hormones produced by the adrenal glands, which is involved in triggering irritability and anger. Cortisol competes with progesterone for receptors that enable progesterone to enter the cells of the body (see page 14). So if your stress levels, and therefore your cortisol levels are high, you may end up with symptoms of progesterone deficiency – even though your body is producing enough.

Secondly, stress may increase the likelihood of PMS by triggering the release of the pituitary hormone prolactin, which stimulates the growth of breast tissue. One of the effects of prolactin (see page 31), is to lower levels of progesterone, which in turn triggers the pituitary to produce more prolactin. This also leads to the effects of progesterone deficiency.

All this may help explain why women in their thirties – one of the most stressful times of life – may be more prone to experience PMS.

Stress and PDD

Research carried out in the United States has found that a faulty biochemical response to stress is likely to be a factor in women suffering from PDD.

Researchers measured levels of a chemical by-product of progesterone called allopregnanolone in the second half of the menstrual cycle. They discovered that healthy women responded to stress by producing more allopregnanolone, while women with PDD produced less. This discovery throws new light on why women with PDD experience such severe symptoms, and could also lead to more effective treatments.

In the genes?

If a woman suffers from PMS, her identical twin is twice as likely to suffer PMS as a non-identical twin or sibling. Daughters whose mothers suffer PMS are also more likely to develop it. Research has also revealed that close relatives of women with PMS are more likely to develop clinical depression. All of this suggests that there could be a genetic tendency towards developing PMS. However, that isn't to say that if your mother had PMS you are bound to suffer it too.

Even if there is a genetic component to PMS, scientists are unlikely to find a single gene that causes it. Rather, as with other common diseases, it is more likely to be a combination of different predisposing genes and their interaction with the environment that brings on PMS.

Childbirth and the pill

Some research has linked having no children or just one child with an increased risk of PMS. This is thought to be because women with fewer pregnancies have more menstrual cycles and are thus exposed more often to cyclical changes in hormone levels. 'PMS is a modern condition,' says Christine Baker of the UK's National Association for Premenstrual Syndrome. 'Since the advent of contraception, smaller families' problems have escalated dramatically, especially with the stressful lives women lead today.'

Research has also shown that women who use the pill as their method of contraception are less likely to have PMS, although coming off the pill may trigger it. The pill irons out fluctuations in hormone levels seen in the natural menstrual cycle which may protect against PMS.

Types of PMS

Because women with PMS report such a puzzling variety of symptoms, in order to make treatment options easier, some experts in the past attempted to categorize PMS according to

Type of PMS	Predominant symptoms
PMS A 'Dr Jekyll and Mr Hyde'	Anxiety: anger, irritability, crying for no reason, verbally and sometimes physically abusive, feeling out of control
PMS D 'Down in the dumps'	Depression: confusion, clumsiness, forgetfulness, withdrawal, fearfulness, paranoia, suicidal thoughts, very occasionally attempted suicide
PMS C 'Carbohydrate cravings'	Cravings: food cravings usually for sweets or chocolate, dairy products including cheese, sometimes alcohol or food in general
PMS H 'Heavy at heart'	Heaviness or headache: fluid retention leading to headache, breast tenderness, abdominal bloating, weight gain

which particular symptoms are predominant. In PMS A, anxiety is the dominant symptom, in PMS D, depression, PMS C, food cravings, and in PMS H, heaviness or headache is the dominant symptom.

The biggest drawback, as every woman with PMS will recognize, is that symptoms rarely fall into such tidy categories. In any case, these groupings are much less used today, with the new understanding of PMS that is emerging. Nevertheless they can be helpful as a way of thinking about your own PMS symptoms and deciding how best to manage them.

Patterns of PMS

Experts have also identified four distinct patterns of PMS, related to the time of the monthly cycle at which a woman experiences symptoms.

❑ Pattern 1: Symptoms begin during the week before your period and recede during your period.

- Pattern 2: Symptoms start around the time of ovulation and carry on until your period starts – that is, for about two weeks.
- Pattern 3: A brief spell of symptoms is experienced around ovulation and then goes away; symptoms recur during the week before menstruation. This pattern often affects teenage girls.
- Pattern 4: Symptoms come on around ovulation and continue over the next weeks and right through menstruation, leaving just a week or ten days without any symptoms.

Whether these patterns relate to an underlying cause is not yet known. Although these groupings may appear to be rather academic, they can be useful in identifying days or weeks when PMS is more likely to be troublesome for you, so that you can take steps to modify your lifestyle, for example, by pacing yourself to avoid stress (see page 53). To establish which pattern your symptoms fall into try keeping a menstrual calendar for two to three months (see page 44).

What are the effects of PMS?

For some women, PMS is little more than a minor nuisance. However, for others it can affect work, relationships and lifestyle, or exacerbate other existing medical conditions (see page 38). For an unfortunate few it comes to dominate their whole existence. For example, some women swell up so much that they need a whole separate set of clothes for the premenstrual period. More seriously, PMS has been cited as a cause of difficulties at home and work, marriage break-up and, in extreme instances, violence and suicide.

Menstrual magnification

Some women with certain chronic conditions experience an exacerbation of symptoms before their period each month. This is known as menstrual magnification. These conditions include medical problems such as arthritis, diabetes and epilepsy, chronic conditions such as Crohn's disease, irritable bowel syndrome, migraine, mental health problems such as depression and eating disorders, and allergies such as asthma, eczema and hayfever. Women may also be more prone to infections including thrush, cystitis, abscesses, skin infections and herpes. What distinguishes menstrual magnification from PMS is that symptoms may be present all the time but they are worse before your period. Even when symptoms aren't physically worsened, if you have a chronic condition you may feel differently about it premenstrually. You may cope perfectly well the rest of the month but feel angry or despairing when you are premenstrual.

Consulting the doctor

If PMS only minimally interferes with your life, you may be able to manage it alone by using some of the self-help methods outlined in the next chapter. However, if your PMS is grinding you down month after month and is seriously disrupting your life and relationships, it is worth seeking medical help.

There are good reasons to see your doctor, apart from simply getting reassurance. In the past, treatment was very hit-and-miss and aimed at controlling symptoms. The discovery of the brain-body links in PMS, however, has led to effective treatments that can improve and sometimes even cure symptoms. They don't work for every woman, but in cases where they do, the relief can be dramatic. There are also a number of other treatments that can help with specific symptoms such as bloating. As well as prescribing medication, your doctor may also be able to help give you practical tips, support and advice on ways to manage your PMS.

Before visiting the doctor

Making a note of the following will help your doctor to diagnose and treat you:

❑ How long you have suffered PMS.

❑ When symptoms first started and any factors associated with this, such as pregnancy or coming off the pill.

❑ Timing of symptoms: when they come on and how long they last. This is where your menstrual calendar can help.

❑ Whether you find that your symptoms are primarily physical or emotional.

❑ Whether your symptoms aggravate other medical conditions (see page 38), for example if you have diabetes whether your blood sugar levels are affected.

❑ Associated symptoms, such as menstrual migraine.

❑ Any self-help measures, complementary treatments or over-the-counter remedies you have tried.

Getting a diagnosis

Before deciding whether you have PMS, the doctor will want to take a full medical history and will ask you questions about your health and lifestyle. These may be about your eating and drinking habits, the amount of exercise you take, the kind of job you do, whether you smoke, whether you are single, cohabiting or married and whether you have children.

There are no specific tests for diagnosing PMS. However, the doctor may want to carry out some investigations to rule out other conditions that could be causing symptoms, such as depression or other emotional problems, an under or overactive thyroid or certain gynaecological disorders. The doctor will also want to check that your symptoms are due to PMS and not menstrual magnification of existing problems (see page 38).

You can help your doctor by keeping a menstrual calendar, which details your symptoms over the course of two or three months. You will find suggestions for how to do this on page 44. The doctor may also want to use a questionnaire or symptom rating scale to monitor your symptoms. If your periods are irregular or your symptoms are erratic, it may be hard to keep a calendar. In this case, the doctor may suggest that you record ovulation (using a temperature chart or hormonal ovulation test kit) to assess its relationship to your symptoms. PMS is only diagnosed if symptoms correlate with the second half of the menstrual cycle.

What the doctor might do

Once he or she has an idea of your symptoms, the doctor will try to evaluate their severity and check whether they are primarily emotional or physical or a mixture of both. If your symptoms are mild to moderate and you are coping quite well, the doctor or nurse will probably advise you on a number of lifestyle measures that can help. You will find details in Chapter 3.

If you have more severe symptoms, the doctor may write you a prescription for one or more of the medications available for treating PMS. You will find a rundown of these in Chapter 4. He or she may also suggest that you visit a PMS clinic if your local hospital has one.

In a few instances, if your symptoms are especially severe or the diagnosis is not clear-cut, the doctor may refer you to a gynaecologist or occasionally a psychiatrist who can investigate you more fully.

Unless you are extremely lucky, it may take a certain amount of trial and error before an appropriate combination of self-management and medication is found. If you are not being helped by a treatment that has been prescribed, don't be afraid to go back to the doctor and ask for further help.

If your doctor isn't helpful

Research carried out by the British National Association for Premenstrual Syndrome (NAPS) suggests that although 66 per cent of doctors do take PMS seriously, around a third of women who visit their doctor find them unsympathetic. Other research shows that over 80 per cent of doctors feel ill-prepared for treating PMS.

It can be extremely demoralizing if, having plucked up the courage to go to the doctor, you feel you are being dismissed. However, don't give up. If your doctor is unhelpful you can ask for a second opinion or change your doctor. If one of the PMS support organizations has a group in your area, they may be able to tell you if there are any doctors locally with a special interest in PMS.

3 Helping yourself

If you have mild to moderate symptoms, you will be pleased to know that there are a host of ways in which you can adjust your lifestyle so as to minimize the effects of PMS. Even if you have severe PMS and your life is seriously disrupted, the self-help measures outlined in this chapter can help reduce your symptoms and make them more manageable.

In this chapter you will find practical, down-to-earth information on helping yourself to cope with PMS. These include looking at your diet, what kind of exercise to take and how to devise an exercise regime that suits you, tips on how to relax and how to get a better night's sleep. You'll also find information on stress management, because anxiety and tension can often exacerbate symptoms, and the importance of getting support so that you don't have to cope alone.

Is it PMS?

The first step you need to take to begin taking control of your PMS is to plot your symptoms on a menstrual calendar. If your symptoms occur regularly after ovulation over two or three cycles, then the chances are that you do have PMS. If, however, your symptoms don't appear to have any particular pattern, occur over the whole month or in the early part of your cycle, then PMS may not be your problem.

Of course you don't have to wait two to three months before putting into action the measures suggested in this chapter. Taking steps to live a healthier, more balanced life will help you feel better anyway – whether or not you have PMS.

Keeping a menstrual calendar

Keeping a menstrual calendar is straightforward. You can either make notes in an ordinary diary or notebook, or draw a chart like the one shown below. Keep your notes handy by your bed, in your handbag, briefcase, or a drawer in your kitchen or office, and get into the habit of making entries at the same time every day. You may want to confine yourself to noting the symptoms that bother you most rather than noting every

MENSTRUAL SYMPTOMS

Day experienced	Details

single symptom, as you may find that this can sometimes be confusing and make it more difficult to detect a pattern during your cycle.

Things to record

❑ The day of your menstrual cycle you experience symptoms. Remember day 1 is the first day of your menstrual flow (proper red blood as opposed to brown blood or spotting).

❑ Details of specific symptoms.

❑ Whether symptoms are mild, moderate or severe – you may like to rate them on a scale of 1–5.

❑ The days of your menstrual period.

As well as your symptoms, make a note of the following, either in the same notebook or diary or on a separate sheet of paper:

❑ What you ate and drank that day.

❑ What kind of sleep you had the night before.

❑ The weather.

❑ Travel activities.

❑ Any exercise you took.

❑ Any chronic conditions you have and their symptoms.

Scale (1–5)	Days of period	Notes

❏ Any medications you took, including over-the-counter or complementary remedies.

❏ Anything else you feel is relevant – perhaps you had a stressful meeting at work, a meeting at your child's school, perhaps you had a row with your partner or went out to a party.

Once you have identified your symptoms and the times when they occur, you will probably see a pattern emerging. You can use this information to begin to fine-tune your lifestyle to minimize the effects of PMS.

Food, diet and alcohol

Improving your diet can do much to help alleviate symptoms. At the end of a busy day, we tend to grab a ready meal from the freezer or order a take-away rather than making a proper meal from fresh ingredients. There is nothing wrong with this from time to time, but if you do it frequently, you could be depriving your body of essential nutrients, which will make your symptoms worse. You will find more details to help you plan your diet in Chapter 6.

Exercise

One of the most beneficial things you can do to relieve PMS is to increase your activity level. The benefits of exercise have been detailed endlessly: better circulation, stronger heart and lungs, more energy and alertness, fewer infections, better mood and sounder sleep.

Numerous studies have proved that people who exercise experience a surge of energy and an uplift in mood that lasts up to an hour after exercising. And several studies have now shown that exercise can specifically help ease PMS. In one study, for example, women put on a programme of regular running experienced a reduction in breast tenderness, fluid retention, depression and stress after just six months, compared with a sedentary group whose symptoms remained the same.

Getting the exercise habit

❏ Start your exercise programme during the early phase of your menstrual cycle when you are feeling more energetic and motivated.

❏ Find ways to incorporate more exercise into your daily life: get off the bus a stop early, walk up stairs rather than taking the lift, throw away the remote control on the TV.

❏ Buy a few exercise and fitness magazines – they're a great source of inspiration and will give you lots of ideas for things you can try at home or at the gym.

❏ Pick an activity you enjoy. Most people can find time for something they like. If you don't enjoy it, you are unlikely to stick at it, especially when you are premenstrual.

❏ Experiment with several different activities at first until you find the one or ones you like best.

❏ Schedule in exercise just like any other activity. If it's down in your diary, you will do it. If you're short of time, consider exercising in the morning before you start work, in the lunch hour or in the evening.

❏ Find ways to motivate yourself. You may find it easier if you join a class or exercise with a friend or partner. Alternatively, you may be someone who prefers to exercise alone or in the comfort of your own home.

- Look for special promotions at your local gym or health club. If you do decide to join a gym, take advantage of the free fitness assessments that are often offered so that your programme is tailored to your individual needs. Tell the instructor you have PMS so that he or she can modify your programme on those days.
- Eat a carbohydrate-rich snack or light meal an hour or so before you exercise to give you energy and help avoid dips in blood sugar which can cause fatigue.
- Be patient: if you do miss the occasional session don't beat yourself up – and don't give up. Simply pick up where you left off the next day.
- On days when you aren't feeling tip-top and don't have the energy for exercise, don't abandon exercise altogether but choose something less strenuous, for example a gentle yoga class rather than power yoga.

Types of exercise

A brisk walk of 15–20 minutes should help lift your mood, but research suggests that for maximum effect you should aim to take 30 minutes of moderate exercise most days. If you aren't used to exercising, this may seem like a lot, so start gently by trying to incorporate more activity into your daily life and build up gradually.

Many women find that once they get the exercise habit they feel so good they don't want to miss a day. On the other hand, some women never positively enjoy exercise, but they keep doing it because they appreciate the benefits of looking and feeling better, having loads more energy and safeguarding their future health.

For total fitness you need to include three types of exercise in your activity programme: aerobic exercise for your heart and lungs, strength exercises for your muscles and stretching exercises for flexibility.

Aerobic exercise

Aerobic exercise is any exercise that gets you sweaty and slightly breathless. It includes cycling, dancing, running, walking and swimming. Aerobic exercise helps condition your heart and lungs. It also helps burn fat and can control premenstrual weight gain and bloating. Aerobic exercise also stimulates the release of the feel-good hormones, known as endorphins. These act like a natural antidepressant to quell depression and mood changes. One study of 23 women with PMS showed that those who took aerobic exercise saw a greater improvement in their symptoms, especially depression, than those who did strength training alone. Aerobic exercise also helps ease fluid retention as it increases circulation and causes you to sweat.

Strength and toning

Resistance or strength training is vital for strong muscles and healthy bones and it's also particularly helpful in reducing the physical symptoms of PMS. You may be worried that building strength will make you look muscular and masculine. This isn't the case: women find it hard to build muscle because they do not have enough of the body-building hormone, testosterone.

What working with weights will do, however, is tone you up, giving you a firmer, more defined shape that will ensure your clothes fit better, even on days when you have put on weight or are bloated. It will also help strengthen your bones, which is especially important to protect against osteoporosis in later life.

Strength training also helps control weight – an important consideration if you have a tendency to gain weight premenstrually. This is because muscle tissue is more metabolically active than other body tissues, and it will continue to burn body fat even when you are sitting still doing absolutely nothing!

To build strength:

❏ Work with fixed-weight machines in a gym or in an exercise studio.

❏ Work with free weights, either at the gym, in a class or at home.

❏ Work with an elasticated exercise band available from sports shops.

❏ Exercise using your own body weight as resistance; for example, try push-ups or abdominal exercises.

❏ Try an exercise system such as yoga or pilates, which uses your body weight to build strength and increase flexibility.

Flexibility and stretching

Flexibility is one of the most vital, yet most neglected, aspects of fitness. Tight muscles limit your ability to move and can lead to injury. When you are flexible, you move with grace and breathe more easily. Daily stretching is the key to becoming flexible: when you stretch, your muscles relax, lengthen and become more elastic. You should always stretch before and after exercising to help prepare your muscles and enable them to recover more quickly. Stretching is also relaxing and

WAYS TO STRETCH

○ Many gyms have instructions for simple stretches posted up on the walls.

○ Aerobics and dance classes should always include five minutes of stretching as part of the warm-up and cool-down. Plié-type exercises are one of the best forms of stretching.

○ Yoga and pilates are both based around stretching, as well as bringing strength and toning benefits.

○ Body work (for example, Thai massage) involves passive stretching – that is, someone else stretches your muscles. This can be especially good on days when you are premenstrual.

○ T'ai chi is an active form of meditation that also includes stretching.

energizing. If you suffer premenstrual fatigue, a few stretches can help banish feelings of tiredness and tension.

Stress management

As we saw in the last chapter, the stressful lives most women lead today have almost certainly contributed to the epidemic of PMS. Research has shown that everyday stresses – such as getting stuck in a traffic jam, the train being late, losing your keys or rushing to get the kids to school – can be more damaging than major stresses such as divorce or bereavement.

Stress is usually a sign that there is some imbalance in your life, so the first step in getting it under control is to take a long, hard look at your life. Some stress is inevitable, of course, but more stress than you can handle can lead to overload and burn-out. Whatever the specific stresses you face, they will be easier to deal with if you are physically fit, rested and eat a nutritious diet. There are also some specific stress-management techniques you can use, to help you when you are premenstrual and at other times of the month.

Everyone's reaction to stress is individual. The important thing to do is to pinpoint those situations you find stressful, and avoid or change them if you can, or find ways to manage your reactions if you cannot.

Beat negative thoughts

Learning to view situations in a more positive light by changing your patterns of thinking can be an enormously helpful step. Psychologists have discovered that people who are depressed or stressed are often perfectionists who think in habitually negative ways that can cause their mood to spiral downwards. Learning to ease up on yourself slightly can break this vicious cycle and cause an upturn in mood.

Planning for stress

Perhaps the greatest secret of stress reduction is to be prepared. Of course there are some stresses you can't avoid, like a sudden bereavement, for example. However, with many stressful situations you can see them coming and take steps to avoid or at least minimize them.

For example, if you're someone who leaves everything to the last minute – anything from setting out for an appointment or meeting to paying your bills on time – life will be more stressful than it would be if you left a bit more time. Try to start allowing twice as much time as you think you are going to need to do something. If necessary, 'trick' yourself into leaving more time by setting all your clocks a quarter of an hour forward. Put your bills on direct debit or standing order to avoid forgetting them, or put a reminder in your diary.

Pacing yourself

An important part of managing PMS is to learn to pace yourself on the days when you are affected. This is where your menstrual calendar (see page 44) comes in useful, because it gives you an idea of the pattern of your PMS. Try to avoid stressful situations when you know you will be premenstrual – for example, if you have the option, put off important meetings until the week after your period, avoid stressful journeys or holidays and try to ease up on your workload. PMS can be a way of your body telling you to slow down and take things a bit easier. If you can accept this rather than trying to fight it, you may find that your symptoms are less troublesome.

Rest and relaxation

When you are stressed, you are more likely to want to drink or smoke to help you relax, you may crave sweets or snacks and be tempted to stop exercising. You feel constantly irritable and worn out.

By contrast, when you are relaxed your breathing slows down, your heart rate and blood pressure are lowered and even your brain waves become smoother. It's possible to induce these changes yourself by learning consciously to relax. There are many different techniques, so pick the one that suits you best.

Ten-minute relaxation

The following is one of the simplest relaxation techniques. You can use it at home or adapt it to your circumstances at work, or even try it on a train or plane.

1 Loosen your belt and any tight clothing, take off your shoes and sit comfortably with your hands resting loosely in your lap. If you are at home you might like to lie down on the floor with a pillow for support under your head and knees.

2 Starting at your toes and working upwards, alternately tense and relax each group of muscles – your feet, calves, thighs, buttocks, abdomen, chest, arms and shoulders, face and scalp. Finally, tense your whole body once and then r-e-l-a-x.

3 Breathe calmly in and out without effort. Don't attempt to force yourself to breathe more deeply. You'll notice that as you become more relaxed your breathing slows and deepens.

4 Stay like this for up to ten minutes. Then stretch in whatever way feels natural to you and get up. Just a short relaxation like this can help ease tension and help you feel much better.

5 If you like you can play a soothing tape or CD while you relax – classical composers rather than the latest heavy-metal band. Alternatively, you might like to use a relaxation or yoga tape.

Ten quick ways to relax

1 Go for a ten-minute walk. Breathe deeply and really notice your surroundings.

2 Get into a good book. Reading is a wonderful way to escape into a different world and forget your own troubles for a time.

3 Sit down for ten minutes with a cup of camomile or lemon balm tea. Drinks like these contain naturally relaxing ingredients.

4 Call a friend. Talking to someone who cares for you is almost guaranteed to make you feel better and will help you to relax.

5 Practise some yoga or pilates or do some stretches.

6 Have a warm bath, to which you have added some calming aromatherapy oils such as lavender, bergamot or neroli, or a mixture of the three.

7 Have a laugh – hire a funny video, read a humorous book, flick to your favourite cartoonist in the newspaper or have a giggle with a friend. Laughter helps ease tension and has been found to have many of the same benefits as more formal relaxation.

8 Stop what you're doing and stand and stare for a few minutes. Noticing the world around you helps take you out of yourself and puts problems into perspective.

9 Put on some uplifting music and dance around the room.

10 Shrug your shoulders and then drop them again and relax. Repeat to yourself a comforting phrase such as 'It doesn't really matter' or 'This too will pass'.

Meditation

Studies of people who meditate regularly have shown that they have lower blood pressure, slower heart rate, better circulation and fewer stress-linked health problems than non-meditators.

There's nothing mysterious about meditation – it's simply a technique for slowing down the incessant chatter of your brain and helping you to relax by concentrating your senses.

There are many different techniques using different senses. Some people like to meditate by focusing on a flower, a lighted candle or an inspiring piece of art work. Others use sound in the form of chanting or singing, or concentrate on a mantra (a word that is repeated endlessly in your head until it loses its meaning). Choose a word that has positive associations for you, such as 'love', 'peace' or the Hindu mantra 'om'. Others visualize a mental scene – a beautiful beach or piece of countryside, or a room – which they enter mentally every time they meditate.

Sit or kneel in an alert but relaxed position and concentrate on your chosen object or sound. If thoughts occur, let them drift across your brain like clouds in the sky. Don't let yourself be hooked by them – just observe them and let them go. It can take a bit of practice to get the knack and some days you may find it easier than others. However, if you persevere you will almost certainly find it helps you to relax and get things into a better perspective.

Sleeping patterns

Sleeping patterns can be disturbed by PMS. Lack of sleep in itself can make you tired, irritable and depressed, causing a particularly vicious cycle. Sleep is very much a habit. Paying attention to getting your sleeping patterns regular (see the suggestions given on page 57) in the early part of your menstrual cycle can help you sleep better before your period, even if you still don't get a perfect night's sleep.

It's also worth taking the opportunity to nap if you aren't sleeping well at night. In fact, research suggests that human beings may actually be programmed to take a siesta, but even if you can't manage a full-blown siesta, mini-naps of ten minutes can be tremendously restorative.

How to encourage a good night's sleep

❑ Try to go to bed at the same time every night so your body clock is programmed to sleep at that time of day. Get up at the same time too – even if you have had a disturbed night. Sleeping late in the morning can lead you to be less sleepy later on.

❑ Make time to wind down in the evening. Play some soothing music or read a relaxing book. Steer clear of action films and stimulating music – you won't be able to sleep if your mind is busy or excited.

❑ Increasing the amount of exercise you get will help you sleep, but avoid vigorous exercise before bedtime. A yoga-type relaxation exercise can help you relax before bed.

❑ Make your bedroom a haven – clear out books, newspapers and the TV. When you are redecorating, use calming colours like blue – avoid red which can be overstimulating.

❑ Make sure your bedroom isn't too hot or cold – ideally it should be 15–18°C (60–65°F). It's better to adjust the temperature by putting on or taking off blankets rather than turning up the central heating.

❑ Avoid eating a heavy meal late at night. However, don't go to bed hungry as low blood sugar can disturb sleep.

❑ A milky drink and a carbohydrate snack before bedtime can help you to sleep better. Tryptophan, an amino acid that is found naturally in foods such as cottage cheese, cashew nuts and turkey, has a natural sedative effect on the body.

❑ Have a warm bath. Raising your body temperature will help make you sleepier.

❑ Cut out tea, coffee, nicotine and other stimulants in the afternoon.

❑ Herb teas such as camomile, lemon balm, hop or valerian contain calming ingredients which can help you get a more restful sleep.

❑ If you do wake in the night and you can't get back to sleep again after about half an hour, don't lie there tossing and turning. Get up and make yourself a soothing camomile tea or a milky drink and do something non-stimulating. Sleep occurs in cycles of around 90 minutes – you'll probably find yourself becoming naturally sleepy again when you hit this point in the cycle.

Seeing the light

The symptoms of PMS are strikingly similar to another syndrome, seasonal affective disorder (SAD), which strikes during the long, dark winter months, affecting women in particular. This has led some researchers to surmise that, like SAD, PMS may be related to a lack of light. Although the exact causes of SAD are not known, it is thought that people with it may produce too much melatonin, a hormone produced in the pea-sized pineal gland in the brain in response to messenger hormones released by the hypothalamus.

Other research suggests that SAD may be linked to lowered levels of neurotransmitters such as serotonin. This makes a lot of sense in view of the fact that the hypothalamus also controls the menstrual cycle and that serotonin and other neurotransmitters are thought to be involved in PMS and PDD. Studies have shown that, in some women with PMS, light treatment helps control symptoms such as cravings, insomnia and depression (see Light Therapy, page 79). At the very least, getting out for a walk in the daylight for an hour or so every day can help lift your mood.

Getting support

When you are plagued with the symptoms of PMS month after month, it's easy to feel alone and as if no one can possibly understand. One of the most valuable ways of helping yourself is simply to talk your feelings over with someone else. Doing so will help you ease feelings of isolation and make you feel more in control of your life.

Provided they are sympathetic, friends and family can be a source of support. Certainly it's a good idea to share how you are feeling with those around you and, if you can, enlist their help for those days when you feel truly awful. However, you may feel that only someone else who has experienced PMS can really understand what you are going through. This is where PMS support groups can be useful. Your doctor or health visitor may be able to tell you if there are any groups locally or you may consider setting up a group yourself.

In recent years with the growth of the Internet and home computers, getting information and support has never been easier. Many health websites have information on PMS – and some have chat rooms where you can talk to other women with PMS at any time of the day or night.

If friends and family aren't sympathetic – indeed, sometimes they may be part of the problem – and if you don't find a support group helpful, you may want to seek professional counselling or psychotherapy – see page 77.

Are there any positive aspects to PMS?

Many women feel there is absolutely nothing positive about their monthly suffering. However, there are some who argue that the character change they undergo during PMS is a source of insight and sometimes even inspiration. Changes in perception that you experience when you have PMS may be indications of an issue in your life that needs to be dealt with. For most of the month you are able to deal with it, but when you have PMS you see things in a different perspective. Some women find it helps to keep a diary when they are premenstrual: writing things down can help dissipate negative emotions, but it can also be a record that you can use at other times of the month to see whether there are any issues you want to deal with.

Another phenomenon that has sometimes been noted is 'premenstrual energy'. Women who write or paint or compose music often say that they have some of their most creative ideas before their period, even though they may not always be able to act on them. The poet Wordsworth defined creativity as 'emotion recollected in tranquillity'. If you can find a way to hang on to the emotion until you are more tranquil – after your period – you may find that there is a way to use the emotional energy creatively.

4 The medical approach

There is a huge and bewildering range of treatments and medications available for treating PMS, probably over 300 in all. This chapter looks at the various medications and supplements that you can get over the counter and on prescription for PMS. It contains information on other kinds of treatment, such as counselling or psychotherapy, or in extreme cases surgery, that your doctor may recommend. It also outlines the most common ways to treat specific symptoms, such as breast pain and swelling, weight gain and bloating, depression, mood swings and headaches.

Treating PMS is not an exact science because its symptoms are variable and rarely clear-cut. There is no panacea and a certain amount of trial and error will usually be needed to discover the best treatment or combination of treatments for you. The exact regimen that your doctor recommends for you is likely to depend on which of your symptoms are predominant, how severe they are and how well they respond to treatment. It will also depend on your doctor's own treatment preferences and his or her judgement as to which treatments are likely to suit you best.

Treatment approaches

Many doctors adopt a stepwise approach to treating premenstrual syndrome, starting with simple lifestyle advice and moving on to more complex or aggressive forms of therapy if these don't work.

The first step is to establish that you do indeed have PMS. The doctor or nurse will then offer you simple advice on diet, exercise, relaxation, stress management and other ways that you can begin to modify your lifestyle. He or she may suggest some simple over-the-counter remedies or vitamin supplementation, or write you a prescription for a simple diuretic (water tablets) or a mild medication such as evening primrose oil to alleviate breast tenderness. He or she may also suggest that you visit a PMS clinic or contact a self-help organization, or refer you for counselling if psychological symptoms are troublesome or if you have other difficulties in your life that are aggravating your PMS.

If your symptoms are mild to moderate, they may well improve by following this regimen. If, after a trial of around three or four months, your symptoms do not improve, the doctor will move on to the second step. The precise treatments vary, but may include prescription medications for the treatment of breast tenderness and other physical symptoms, hormonal medications or antidepressant drugs of the SSRI (selective serotonin reuptake inhibitor) group for psychological symptoms such as mood swings, depression and food cravings.

If you're one of the unlucky few whose symptoms don't respond to these measures in step two, the doctor will move on to step three. This will usually involve referring you to a specialist who may prescribe medication for around six months which suppresses the hormones that trigger ovulation. In effect, this triggers an artificial menopause. For this reason, the doctor may also prescribe other drugs, such as hormone replacement therapy (HRT), to prevent menopausal symptoms and to protect your bones. In rare instances, if all else fails, the specialist may recommend a hysterectomy with removal of the ovaries. In this case you will be offered HRT to prevent menopausal symptoms, such as hot flushes, and to protect your bones from the effects of early menopause.

The stepwise approach

Step One: mild to moderate symptoms Lifestyle advice and support, such as a healthy diet, exercise, nutritional supplements and stress management; pulsed light treatment (photic stimulation); over-the-counter medications or mild prescription medications for breast pain or bloating.

Step Two: moderate to severe symptoms Hormonal treatments, such as progesterone for physical and emotional symptoms, the contraceptive pill or oestrogen patches; antidepressants of the SSRI group for mood symptoms; stronger prescribed medications for breast tenderness and other specific symptoms.

Step Three: severe symptoms Drugs that suppress your natural menstrual cycle; hysterectomy with removal of the uterus and ovaries to induce early menopause; hormone replacement therapy (HRT) to prevent menopausal symptoms and effects.

Over-the-counter options

There are a host of over-the-counter preparations that you can buy in the pharmacy or health food shop for treating PMS. Your doctor may suggest one or more of these. Alternatively, if your PMS is mild or moderate, you may like to try them to see if they help alleviate symptoms. The pharmacist can help you decide which ones are likely to be most helpful.

If you find that you are not being helped by these treatments after giving them a trial of, say, three or four months, or if you experience unpleasant side effects, you should stop taking them and see your doctor to discuss alternative options. It's important to inform your doctor and pharmacist if you are taking any over-the-counter medications, even 'natural' treatments such as vitamin or mineral supplements and herbal remedies.

When buying medications over the counter, you need to take just as much care as you would if you were prescribed them by a doctor. Just because a medication is available over the counter, it doesn't mean that it can't be harmful if used incorrectly. It's especially important to check with the pharmacist if you are taking medication for another condition or if you suspect that you might be pregnant. You should also pay close attention to labelling. Some medications contain several active ingredients when in fact a simple medication with just one might be sufficient to alleviate your symptoms. Generally, the more simple it is, the better. Always read and follow the instructions on the packet and never take more than the stated dose. Bear in mind that over-the-counter medications can only provide relief – they won't cure the symptoms of PMS.

Analgesics

Certain analgesic or painkilling drugs work by blocking or reducing the production of prostaglandins, chemicals which help pass on pain signals to the brain and are involved in controlling the process of inflammation in the body. They include aspirin, ibuprofen and other medications belonging to the non-steroidal anti-inflammatory drugs (NSAID) group of medications. They can be useful for quelling abdominal cramps, headaches and migraine and breast pain.

Watchpoints

❑ Avoid aspirin if you have peptic ulcers or other digestive problems. It should not be used by anyone with a bleeding disorder or anyone with asthma or long-term kidney or liver problems.

❑ Do not use ibuprofen if you have long-term kidney problems, high blood pressure, asthma, peptic ulcers or other digestive disorders. It should also be avoided if you have ever had an allergic reaction to aspirin.

❑ Taking these antiprostaglandin medications with food may help avoid digestive upsets.

❑ Both aspirin and ibuprofen should be avoided if you think you are pregnant, except on the advice of your doctor.

Diuretics (water tablets)

Many mild diuretics are on sale at the pharmacy. There are also a number of herbal diuretics containing herbs such as parsley, celery seed and shepherd's purse, which are available from health food stores.

Diuretics are used to promote the flow of urine by increasing the work of the kidneys. They are used to treat fluid retention. At one time they were widely used to treat PMS, but they are less popular today. In fact, many experts believe they have no real place in the treatment of PMS. Diuretics can leach both potassium and magnesium from the body, both of which are involved in helping maintain the body's fluid balance, so taking them can be counterproductive.

Watchpoints

❑ Diuretics may upset the body's mineral balance – in particular of potassium. Given that a shortage of minerals may be a factor in PMS, they are probably best avoided.

❑ Newer potassium-sparing diuretics avoid this problem. However, there is no good evidence that they are useful in PMS.

❑ A low-salt diet and drinking plenty of water are probably the best ways to help control fluid retention and bloating.

GLA supplements
(evening primrose oil, starflower (borage) oil, blackcurrant seed oil)

These all contain omega-6 fatty acids, which are converted in the body into gamma-linolenic acid (GLA). GLA is needed for the production of hormone-like substances called prostaglandins, which are necessary for the healthy functioning of cells. A key role of prostaglandins is to render certain cells, in particular breast cells, less sensitive to the effects of female hormones.

Some experts believe that a major cause of PMS is the body's inability to convert omega-6 into GLA. GLA synthesis can be reduced by a number of factors, including transfatty acids (found in dairy foods, pastries, biscuits, cakes and other processed foods and margarines) and too much alcohol. Although studies haven't always been conclusive, there is evidence that evening primrose oil (the most tested of the GLA supplements) can ease breast pain.

Watchpoints

❏ A dose of three or four 500 mg evening primrose oil capsules a day for at least four months is recommended. If pain is alleviated, you can reduce the dose to one capsule a day. If you don't experience relief after four months, see the doctor.

❏ Evening primrose oil is generally safe but side effects can include bloating, depression, diarrhoea, headaches, nausea, stomach upsets and rashes.

❏ Don't take evening primrose oil if you suffer from any form of epilepsy.

St John's Wort

St John's Wort (*Hypericum perforatum*) is a herbal remedy that has been used for centuries for the treatment of depression, inflammation and anxiety. In the past few years, it has been hailed as a kind of natural antidepressant because it is believed it may act in the same way as antidepressants of the SSRI group to raise levels of the brain chemical, serotonin. A number of research studies have shown St John's Wort to be as effective as some antidepressants in treating mild to moderate depression and depressive symptoms of PMS.

Watchpoints

❑ It can take two or three weeks for effects to be felt, so be patient and persevere.

❑ St John's Wort seems to have remarkably few side effects, the main one being mild stomach upset. However, animals grazing on large amounts of St John's Wort may become allergic to sunlight, so it may be wise to avoid sun exposure while you are taking it, especially if you have a fair skin.

❑ Avoid taking St John's Wort if you are already taking prescribed antidepressants.

❑ Don't take St John's Wort if you are pregnant or breastfeeding.

❑ Always let your doctor and pharmacist know if you are taking St John's Wort, as there may be interactions with other medications.

Vitamin and mineral supplements

Research suggests that women with PMS may be short of one or more of a number of vitamins and minerals. As well as those detailed below, there are multivitamin and mineral supplements specifically formulated for PMS. Research indicates that some of these can have a positive effect in alleviating the symptoms of PMS.

There's a tendency to think that because vitamins and minerals are found naturally in food that they are harmless. This is far from being the case. Vitamins and minerals are pharmacologically active, which means that they change the chemistry of your body cells. In addition, many vitamins and minerals are synergisetic, meaning that they work together. So while the vitamins and minerals found in a carrot, apple or banana, for example, are perfectly balanced, taking them in isolation in a food supplement could cause dietary imbalances. For example, all the B vitamins work together, as do vitamin B6 and magnesium, so if you are taking a B6 supplement, you need to make sure your diet is rich in other B vitamins and contains some magnesium-rich foods too. Some supplements can interfere with the action of certain drugs. For example, high doses of vitamin D or calcium ascorbate should be avoided if you taking the heart medication digoxin.

It is worth reading the labels to make sure you know what you are buying as some cheaper supplements are padded out with fillers. As a rule, you get what you pay for, although buying them by phone or over the Internet may save you money. Unless you are simply planning to take a multi-vitamin or mineral it's a good idea to consult a nutritional therapist.

Vitamin B6 (pyridoxine)

B vitamins are needed to help the liver metabolize the female sex hormone oestrogen, thus lowering its level in the bloodstream before a period. Vitamin B6 itself has a long and rather chequered history. However, a number of studies have found that it can help improve symptoms such as mood swings, breast tenderness and headaches.

B6 is essential for the manufacture of the brain chemicals serotonin and dopamine, key culprits in the mood changes of PMS. It also plays a role in the synthesis of prostaglandins and works closely with magnesium, which is needed for serotonin production in the body.

Until 1998, supplements of B6 were often recommended for the treatment of premenstrual syndrome. However, in that year, following reports that the high doses could damage the central nervous system, the UK government issued an edict that doses of over 10 mg should only be used under medical supervision. Currently this has been suspended awaiting further trials. The current recommendation is 50–100 mg of B6 a day plus 250 mg of magnesium.

Watchpoints
❑ Taking the contraceptive pill may increase the body's need for B6.
❑ Take B6 with food to avoid stomach upset.
❑ High doses are potentially toxic to the nerves. If you experience tingling in the hands and feet, stop taking B6 and consult your doctor.

Calcium
Calcium is the most abundant mineral in the body. As well as its best-known role in maintaining strong bones and teeth, calcium also helps aid the transmission of chemical messages within the brain.

A shortage of calcium (hypocalcaemia) is associated with low mood, depression and anxiety, symptoms that mirror those of PMS. It is known that female sex hormones influence the way the body deals with calcium. In fact, studies have found that women with PMS who take a calcium supplement experience fewer mood swings and symptoms such as anxiety, irritability, anger and tearfulness.

Calcium works best when taken with vitamin D, sometimes called the sunshine vitamin because the body metabolizes it from sunlight on the skin. Taken together in the order of 1000 mg a day of calcium and 10 mcg of vitamin D, they can help treat premenstrual cramps, backache and migraine and some of the emotional symptoms of PMS.

Watchpoints

❑ Ask your pharmacist for 'chelated' calcium – chelation is a chemical process that makes calcium easier to absorb.

❑ Too little magnesium in the diet disrupts calcium metabolism (see below).

❑ Calcium can interfere with the effectiveness of the antibiotic tetracycline. Make sure that you tell your doctor if you are taking calcium.

Magnesium

Magnesium is the second most abundant mineral inside our body's cells and is sometimes known as the anti-stress mineral. Studies have shown that women who suffer from PMS often have low levels of magnesium. Use of the contraceptive pill and a high alcohol intake are also associated with magnesium deficiency.

Magnesium may play a role in PMS in several ways. Firstly, it works in harmony with vitamin B6 to synthesize GLA in the body (see page 66). Secondly, it is needed for the metabolism of brain chemicals, the proper function of the adrenals and for converting glucose into energy – all of which may play a part in PMS. Thirdly, a lack of magnesium may be a factor in bloating and swelling, as it pushes up levels of an adrenal hormone, aldosterone, which is responsible for regulating the excretion of salt by the kidneys and hence the body's fluid balance. Diuretics can lower magnesium levels, creating a vicious cycle.

Several research studies have shown a beneficial effect from taking magnesium for a range of PMS symptoms including migraine, mood swings and anxiety.

Watchpoints

❏ Supplements should not be taken after meals, as magnesium neutralizes stomach acidity and interferes with digestion.
❏ Some doctors advise supplementation of 250 mg a day with 50–100 mg of vitamin B6 for optimum effectiveness.
❏ If no improvement is seen after four months, stop taking it and consult your doctor.
❏ Side effects are few, but taking too much magnesium may cause diarrhoea.

Zinc

Many women who suffer with PMS symptoms are deficient in zinc, a mineral that directs and oversees the efficient flow of many body processes, including the formation of insulin and certain aspects of brain function. It also helps skin healing and has, along with vitamin A, been found to be useful in the treatment of premenstrual acne.

Watchpoints

❑ For treating acne, the recommended dose is 7 mg a day, coupled with 600 mcg a day of vitamin A.

❑ High levels of vitamin A have been associated with birth defects, and should be avoided if you are planning a pregnancy or could get accidentally pregnant.

Prescription treatments

If the measures previously outlined don't help with your symptoms, there are a number of treatments that your doctor can prescribe for you. They include hormonal treatments (see below) that alter or suppress the menstrual cycle, talking treatments, and a number of treatments for specific premenstrual symptoms.

It's important to work with your doctor so that, together, you can decide on the most appropriate treatment for you. When the doctor gives you a prescription, make sure you know exactly what medication is being prescribed and why. You should also know exactly how and when to take it and what side effects you might experience. If you do experience side effects, don't be afraid to go back to the doctor. He or she may be able to prescribe a different medication or alter the dosage.

Progesterone

The theory that some women with PMS need larger-than-average amounts of progesterone was proposed by British endocrinologist Dr Katharina Dalton as long ago as the 1940s. Dalton found that treating women with natural progesterone (as opposed to the synthetic form) helped alleviate symptoms such as aggression, anxiety, bloating, breast tenderness, irritability, lowered mood and panic attacks. Millions of women over the years have testified to the beneficial effects of progesterone. However, recent research has failed to confirm its efficacy and many doctors feel that its benefits are not sufficiently proven.

Progesterone is destroyed in the body by the liver, so it cannot be taken by mouth. Instead it is prescribed in the form of pessaries, which are inserted into the rectum or the vagina. It can also be administered in the form of a vaginal cream. Occasionally, if other methods of administration don't bring relief, it can be given by injection.

Watchpoints

- ❏ May alter the length of your menstrual cycle and cause diarrhoea and wind.
- ❏ Some women using progesterone report developing acne and changes in libido.
- ❏ Can cause pregnancy symptoms, such as nausea and swollen breasts.
- ❏ Avoid pessaries or gel coming into contact with barrier contraceptives.
- ❏ Pessaries can worsen vaginal thrush. If you are prone to thrush, tell your doctor who will probably suggest that you use pessaries rectally rather than vaginally.
- ❏ Injections of progesterone can cause bruising of muscle tissue and soreness.
- ❏ Progesterone should not be used if you suffer from abnormal vaginal bleeding or have a history of blood-clotting disorders. Caution is also needed if you have liver dysfunction.

Progestogen

Progestogen is the synthetic form of progesterone used in many contraceptive pills and HRT preparations. There are several different brands of tablets, and it is also used in a progestogen IUD (intra-uterine device for contraception).

Some clinical trials have shown progestogen to be effective in treating the symptoms of PMS. However, some women find that it causes side effects of the very same kind as the symptoms they are prescribed to treat, although these usually ease over time.

Watchpoints

❑ Side effects may include stomach upsets and skin disorders, breast pain, lactation, abnormal menstrual bleeding and weight gain.

❑ Other potential side effects may include acne, fluid retention, changes in libido, irregular periods, mood changes and insomnia.

❑ Caution is needed if you have diabetes, epilepsy, migraine, asthma and heart or kidney failure.

The combined pill

The combined pill ('the pill') contains oestrogen and progestogen. Some women's symptoms improve when they are on the pill because it stops ovulation. However, women who are sensitive to their own hormones may be sensitive to the synthetic hormones used in the pill. In addition, coming off the pill is frequently a trigger for PMS. The pill seems most effective for physical symptoms of PMS. Triphasic pills, which contain varying amounts of hormones according to the stage of your cycle, have been found to be more effective than monophasic ones, which contain fixed amounts of hormone in each pill.

Watchpoints

❑ Side effects can include breast tenderness, dizziness, headaches, mood changes, nausea and weight gain. These usually disappear within three months. If they don't, changing the type of pill may help.

❑ In rare instances, the pill can cause blood clots that block a blood vessel (thrombosis).

❑ If you are obese, have severe varicose veins, smoke, have diabetes, high blood pressure or a history of venous thrombosis, heart attack or stroke at an early age in your immediate family, you may be at an increased risk of thrombosis. If you think you may be at risk, discuss with your doctor whether the pill is right for you.

Oestrogen patches and implants

Oestrogen has a chemical effect on mood. In studies of post-menopausal women on HRT, oestrogen has been found to alleviate irritability, fatigue, anxiety, depression and poor memory. Other studies show that it improves sleep.

Oestrogen patches used twice weekly have been found to be effective in controlling mood symptoms in many women with PMS. These are small, transparent sticky 'plasters' containing oestrogen, which you stick on to the skin of the abdomen or upper thigh. Oestrogen implants, tiny pellets which are inserted under the skin to release oestrogen gradually into the bloodstream, may also be used.

Oestrogen therapies work by suppressing ovulation and ironing out fluctuations of hormones. Like any kind of HRT, oestrogen cannot be given alone, except to women who have had a hysterectomy. This is because it causes a build-up of the uterine lining (the endometrium), raising the risk of cancer of the uterus or endometrium. For this reason, progestogen or progesterone has to be given as well, to cause the body to slough off the endometrium.

Watchpoints
❑ Side effects of oestrogen include breast pain, nausea and weight gain. Progestogen or progesterone can also cause unwanted side effects (see pages 74 and 75).

Treatments for psychological symptoms

With treatments for mood problems, more so than physical symptoms, your attitude can play a significant role in the effectiveness of a treatment. Research has shown that psychotherapy can be useful on its own or combined with medication, so if you would prefer to try counselling to anti-depressant drugs, for example, it's worth telling your doctor. You should still try to keep an open mind, however. There may be instances in which taking an anti depressant can lift your mood sufficiently to enable you to tackle your problems more constructively. Whatever treatment you decide upon, the doctor will usually want to reassess you after a period of time.

Selective serotonin reuptake inhibitors (SSRIs)

The treatment of the psychological symptoms of PMS has been revolutionized in the past few years with the advent of a new group of antidepressants which act by raising levels of the brain hormone serotonin. These include fluoxetine and paroxetine. SSRIs are less sedating and are better tolerated than the older tricyclic antidepressants, which were not effective in PMS. Research suggests that 60–70 per cent of women with severe PMS experience a significant reduction in symptoms. Fluoxetine has been shown to be especially effective for PDD.

SSRIs seem to kick into action much more quickly (within one to two days) when used to treat PMS-linked mood problems than when used for other types of depression. The doctor may prescribe an SSRI to be used throughout your menstrual cycle or just during the last couple of weeks.

Watchpoints

❑ Stomach upsets are the most common side effects. Other side effects can include tiredness, nervousness, dizziness and difficulty concentrating. These usually ease within a few weeks.

❑ SSRIs should be used with caution if you have epilepsy, diabetes, bleeding disorders, liver or kidney impairment, or if you are pregnant or breastfeeding.

❑ Never suddenly stop taking an SSRI – phase out slowly.

Talking treatments

If depression or mood symptoms are a prominent feature of your PMS, or you have menstrual magnification of an existing mood disorder, the doctor may recommend counselling or psychotherapy.

One type of psychotherapy that is often particularly useful is cognitive therapy, which is based on the idea that the way we think affects how we feel. Cognitive therapy has consistently been found to be as successful as antidepressants for the treatment of mild and moderate depression.

In a cognitive therapy session, the therapist helps you to pinpoint your thoughts and test them against reality. You are then taught to change unrealistic or distorted thoughts to more positive and realistic ones. Changing the way you think can have a dramatic effect on the way you feel, often in quite a short span of time. Your doctor may be able to recommend a local therapist.

Watchpoints

❑ Before you begin treatment, check how many sessions you are likely to require and how long they last.

❑ Any form of psychotherapy or counselling will work best if you are committed to it.

❑ Before starting, think about what you want from the therapy. Consider not just your PMS symptoms but any other areas of your life.

Light therapy (photic stimulation)

The effect of light on our health has long been known, and the role of light treatment for the symptoms of seasonal affective disorder (SAD) is well established. Photic stimulation is a type of light therapy which uses coloured or pulsed light. Miniature lamps mounted on a light mask similar to a pair of sunglasses are used to deliver doses of gently pulsed light for 15 minutes a day during the second half of the menstrual cycle. In a research study, the treatment reduced symptoms by 76 per cent in 17 women with PMS. The treatment was particularly useful for depression and mood swings, but women in the study also reported improvements in the symptoms of period pains, sleep and food cravings.

Watchpoints

❑ Caution is needed because, although the trial mentioned had remarkable results, it was not a blind trial – the women knew they were receiving treatment, so there may have been a placebo effect.

❑ Photic stimulation has also been found to reduce migraine and you may find this treatment useful if you suffer with premenstrual migraine.

Treatments for breast swelling and pain

The main medical treatments for breast swelling and pain are powerful hormonal drugs which can have quite dramatic side effects. For this reason, unless breast pain and swelling are making your life a complete misery, you should think carefully before taking them and find out if there are other, simpler measures that might be more helpful. If you do decide to take these medications, you should discuss the implications in detail with your doctor.

Danazol

Danazol is a powerful drug used to suppress ovulation. It is used to treat endometriosis and fibrocystic breast disease (the tendency to lumpy breasts which is often exacerbated by PMS). Danazol can be effective for premenstrual breast pain, but has side effects that generally make it a poor choice for treatment (see above).

Watchpoints

❑ Side effects include voice deepening and hair growth which may be irreversible.

❑ It can also cause lack of periods, weight gain, decreased breast size, acne and fluid retention.

❑ Other side effects include hot flushes, vaginal dryness and mood swings. Long-term therapy can affect blood fat levels and bone density.

❑ Danazol should not be used in pregnancy, so if you are prescribed it, use a non-hormonal method of contraception just in case you become pregnant.

Bromocriptine

Bromocriptine, a drug sometimes used to dry up milk in women who don't want to breastfeed, works to reduce prolactin levels, which as we've seen are thought by some to be a factor in PMS. It's been reported to be helpful in reducing severe breast pain and tenderness.

Watchpoints

❑ Side effects of bromocriptine can include dizziness, headaches, fatigue and nausea.

Treatments for weight gain and bloating

The most common medical treatment for weight gain and bloating are diuretics, drugs that increase the amount of fluid excreted by your kidneys and, in consequence, decrease fluid and the salt (sodium) levels in the body. Used as prescribed, they are generally pretty safe, but if you take too many of them, they can upset the body's mineral balance, so it's important always to take only the dose that has been prescribed by your doctor.

Diuretics

Diuretics used to be a mainstay of PMS treatment, because it was believed that they acted to rid the body of excess oestrogen. This theory is now discredited. However, diuretics may still be prescribed to help ease bloating and weight gain, although research suggests that only women who actually pile on pounds premenstrually really benefit. Spironolactone, a potassium-sparing diuretic (see page 66), may be prescribed by the doctor.

Watchpoints

❑ Potassium depletion can be a side effect of some diuretics especially if you are also restricting your salt intake.

❑ Ask your doctor about whether you should take a potassium supplement and make sure you eat plenty of potassium-rich foods, such as bananas, tomatoes, oranges and dried fruit.

❑ Some diuretics may raise cholesterol or blood sugar levels in the body. Remind your doctor if you have diabetes or a heart condition.

Treatments that suppress ovarian function

If your PMS is so severe that the treatments outlined so far don't help, the doctor may decide to use more aggressive methods of stopping ovulation and thus removing your menstrual cycle. This can be done either with drugs or, extremely rarely, by hysterecomy, the surgical removal of your uterus and the ovaries.

GnRH analogues

GnRH analogues are drugs that suppress the natural menstrual cycle and are also used to stop ovulation before fertility treatments such as IVF (in vitro fertilization – the test tube technique). They are given by nasal spray or injection. In effect they mimic the menopause and because of this they are not suitable for long-term use. They will only be prescribed for a maximum of six months, because of the risk of menopausal effects such as osteoporosis. If you are going to take GnRH analogues the doctor will also prescribe HRT or a drug called tibolone, which prevents hot flushes and protects against osteoporosis.

Watchpoints

❑ PMS symptoms may be exacerbated during the first month of treatment, so be patient and persevere.

❑ Side effects can include hot flushes, headaches, muscle aches, vaginal dryness and mood swings.

❑ GnRH analogues should not be used in pregnancy, so you should use a non-hormonal method of contraception such as the cap, condom or IUD to prevent you from becoming pregnant.

❑ Although it is possible that GnRH analogue treatment can reduce PMS, it may not be effective for women with severe PDD or menstrual magnification of depression and other mood disorders.

Surgery

If all else fails, and very much as a last resort, the doctor may recommend the removal of your uterus, ovaries and Fallopian tubes, an operation known medically as hysterectomy with bilateral salpingo-oophorectomy (BSO), to induce an early menopause. This is a drastic and controversial solution that you will want to think very carefully about before going ahead.

HRT will be prescribed to alleviate menopausal effects. After the uterus has been removed, oestrogen alone can be given and progestogen will not be necessary.

Watchpoints

❏ Try to get as much information as possible before you make a decision. Contact a support group and talk your decision over with friends and family.

❏ As with any surgery, there are some risks associated with the anaesthestic and the operation itself. These can include haemorrhage, damage to the bladder, cystitis and, rarely, development of a blood clot in the leg veins (venous thrombosis).

❏ After the operation you will need to take it easy and you will need help with childcare, household tasks, shopping and anything that involves lifting and carrying.

❏ Some women experience an adverse effect on their sex lives. However, others find the improvement in symptoms brings such relief that the reverse is true.

5 Complementary treatments

Several complementary therapies may be beneficial in PMS, including acupuncture and acupressure, aromatherapy, herbal medicine, homoeopathy, massage and reflexology. No one therapy stands out as being particularly beneficial for PMS, although research is looking at both Western and Chinese herbal treatments and acupuncture with some extremely promising results.

One of the things many women value is the way in which complementary practitioners view health and disease. They believe that good health is the body's natural condition and that anything else is a deviation from this. There is also an emphasis, not always seen in orthodox medicine, on taking responsibility for your own health, rather than simply handing over your symptoms to a doctor and waiting for a cure. This makes complementary medicine useful for a condition like PMS, where many women report feeling out of control. Above all, many complementary therapies are supremely relaxing and, given the connection with stress, this is important. Women with PMS often say that, even if symptoms are not completely banished, they feel better able to cope with them.

Herbal medicine

Herbal medicine has been the origin of a number of treatments that have now passed into mainstream medicine. Among the most well-known, at least as far as PMS is concerned, are evening primrose oil, which is now a well-accepted prescription medication for the treatment of premenstrual breast pain and tenderness, and St John's Wort, used to treat the depressive symptoms of PMS (see page 67).

Herbalism involves using plants, flowers, trees and herbs to stimulate the body's own self-healing mechanism. Herbs have always been, and still are, used throughout the world. In fact, it has been estimated by the World Health Organization (WHO) that 80 per cent of people in the world today still rely on herbs as their primary medicine.

Herbal remedies are used to support the body as it heals itself and also to prevent disease from recurring. Despite extensive research and analysis, scientists have still been unable to pinpoint every chemical component of herbs. They have, however, discovered that herbs contain vitamins, minerals, carbohydrates, trace elements and a number of other plant chemicals that have healing properties.

The various herbal traditions have thrown up a number of useful treatments for PMS and an increasing amount of

HERBAL REMEDIES FOR SPECIFIC SYMPTOMS

Symptoms	Useful herbs
Digestion and control of blood sugar	Gentian
Anxiety and tension	Oats, Skullcap, Camomile, Valerian
Migraine	Feverfew
Bloating and fluid retention	Dandelion tea
Abdominal cramps	Raspberry leaf tea, Camomile, Cramp bark
Headaches	Ginger
Nausea associated with migraine	Cinnamon, Ginger

research is being done into their use. Several herbs have been subject to clinical research studies of the kind used to test orthodox drugs, although they are not always as well-controlled as orthodox trials.

Vitex agnus-castus (chaste tree, hemp tree, monk's pepper)

One herb that has been studied lately as a treatment for PMS is Vitex agnus-castus, a plant that has been traditionally used to alleviate symptoms of PMS. It contains a mixture of plant chemicals and compounds similar in structure to the female sex hormones. Scientists surmise that it may work in a similar way to the corpus luteum, which is produced in the luteal phase of the menstrual cycle. It may also help modulate the secretion of prolactin, the hormone that has been implicated in PMS, so increasing progesterone. In a large controlled European trial reported in the prestigious *British Medical Journal* in January 2001, Vitex agnus-castus tablets were found to be more effective than a placebo in quelling most symptoms of PMS, including irritability, mood swings, anger, headaches and painful, swollen breasts.

Watchpoints

❑ Possible side effects include stomach upsets, itching, rashes, hair loss, headaches and fatigue.

❑ Caution is needed with certain drugs, including metoclopramide and the contraceptive pill.

Cimicifuga racemosa (black cohosh, baneberry, black snakeroot, bugbane, rattleroot)

This is a native North American plant, historically used for menstrual and menopausal disturbances, whose roots and rhizome contain a number of active plant chemicals with an oestrogen-like effect.

Black cohosh is used by the body to make progesterone. It also contains salicylic acid, the prime component of aspirin, which has anti-inflammatory and pain-relieving properties. Although primarily useful for treating menopausal problems, its pain-relieving qualities may make it a helpful remedy for PMS symptoms such as abdominal cramps, headaches and breast pain.

Watchpoints

❑ Side effects can include nausea, vomiting, dizziness and disturbances of the nervous system and eyesight.

❑ It may interact with other salicylic acid-containing drugs and herbs, and anticoagulants (which stop blood clotting).

Angelica sinensis (dong quai)

Dong quai is the female medicine *par excellence* in traditional Chinese medicine. It has been found to contain vitamin B12, a shortage of which is implicated in PMS. It also contains ferrulic acid, a painkiller and other compounds that act to relax or stimulate the uterus. It is used for abdominal cramps, irregular periods and other problems linked to menstruation.

Watchpoints

❑ Dong quai can cause sun sensitivity or a sun-induced rash. For this reason you should avoid sunlight when you are taking it.

❑ You should also avoid herbs or medications that cause increased bleeding or affect blood clotting.

Piper methysticum (kava kava, awa, kew, tonga and wurzelstock)

Kava kava, which derives from a Hawaiian word meaning bitter, has been known in the Pacific for centuries and is used in a ceremonial drink used to settle disputes, celebrate marriage and welcome visitors. A perennial shrub and a member of the pepper family, piper methysticum has natural tranquillizing and sedative properties.

This herbal remedy works by acting on the body's limbic system, which helps control emotion. Several studies have found piper methysticum to be effective in reducing anxiety, without experiencing the drowsiness and difficulty of operating machinery that may be found in other more conventional tranquillizers.

Watchpoints

❑ Side effects can include stomach upsets, headaches, dizziness and rashes.

❑ Stop using if problems are persisting.

❑ Caution should be used if taking other medications or herbs that act on the central nervous system.

Valeriana officinalis (valerian)

A strong relaxant and antispasmodic, valerian has been used since the 18th century to treat insomnia and nervous problems where anxiety predominates. Its active ingredient is a compound that blocks the breakdown of a chemical called gamma-aminobutyric acid. This decreases central nervous system activity. Several studies have shown that it reduces the length of time it takes to drop off at night (sleep latency) and improves quality of sleep, especially in young women and poor sleepers. Valerian can also be used for abdominal cramps, constipation due to irritable bowel, headaches, migraine and sciatica.

Watchpoints

❑ Side effects can include morning sleepiness, headache, excitability, anxiety and, ironically, insomnia.

❑ It should not be used indefinitely and should not be used with other medications or herbs with sedative effects.

Other therapies

A whole host of other complementary therapies can help PMS including acupuncture, aromatherapy, homeopathy, massage and reflexology. No one treatment is best, so it's largely a matter of trial and error to find one that helps you. As always when visiting a complementary therapist, it's important to find someone with whom you feel comfortable. Personal recommendation is often a good way to find a complementary therapist. However, you should always check that the therapist is properly qualified and ask if he or she has experience of treating PMS and with what results. The therapist should give you some idea of how long you will need to have therapy and how long it will be before you can expect to experience an improvement in symptoms.

Acupuncture and acupressure

Acupuncture is one of the most ancient complementary therapies. It originated in China over 5,000 years ago and today, according to the World Health Organization (WHO), is effective in the treatment of over 40 disorders, including PMS. Acupuncture and acupressure is part of the much broader discipline of traditional Chinese medicine, which includes Chinese herbalism, moxibustion, massage, dietary therapy and meditative exercise such as T'ai chi.

According to traditional Chinese theory, our bodies have more than 2,000 acupuncture points placed along twelve main and eight secondary pathways called meridians. Chinese practitioners believe these meridians channel energy (*chi* or *qi*) between the surface of the body and its internal organs.

Chi is the body's vital energy which supports, nourishes and defends us against mental, physical and emotional disease. Blood can be a form of *chi*. If the flow of *chi* is blocked, stagnated or weakened, ill health results. A smooth flow of *chi* is dependent on a balance of two opposing forces known as yin and yang. Traditionally, yin is the dark, passive, feminine, cold and negative force, while yang is light, active, male, warm and positive. Acupuncture is believed to work by balancing yin and yang and so restoring the flow of *chi*. Acupressure works in a similar way, except that, instead of using needles, finger pressure is used on the acupuncture points.

Although doctors have failed so far to accommodate Chinese theory within the framework of Western medicine, there are suggestions that acupuncture may work by stimulating the central nervous system to release messenger chemicals such as neurotransmitters. These act on the brain to quell pain or to release other chemicals, such as endorphins (the body's feel-good hormones) and other hormones, which stimulate the body's regulatory mechanisms, so restoring the body to a state of balance.

In the light of recent theories about PMS and the role of neurotransmitters, it would make a great deal of sense that acupuncture is an effective treatment and, in fact, several studies have shown that it can help rebalance hormones and alleviate symptoms. According to Chinese medicine, PMS is a result of faulty liver function which, according to Chinese belief, leads to stagnation of *chi*.

Aromatherapy

Aromatherapy involves the use of essential oils in a number of treatments to improve health and emotional wellbeing and restore the body to balance. Essential oils are derived from the bark, leaves, fruit and seeds of plants, flowers and trees. Around 150 essential oils exist, each with its own unique aroma and healing properties.

Essential oils can be used in a number of ways – in inhalations, diffusers and vaporizers, in baths, compresses and in massage. It's not known exactly how aromatherapy oils work, but it could have something to do with the fact that the hormones and messenger chemicals found in plants interact in some way with the hormones and messenger chemicals within the human body. However they work, aromatherapy can have a striking effect, both on physical symptoms and the emotions.

For PMS, try the following treatments:

- ❑ Use a few drops of clary sage, geranium and lavender in the bath, to uplift, calm and ease fatigue.
- ❑ Try cold lavender compresses for tender, painful breasts.
- ❑ Geranium, bergamot and rosemary massage is good for treating tiredness and lethargy.
- ❑ A head and neck massage using lavender oil can clear headaches and migraine.
- ❑ Inhale sandalwood and camomile to alleviate stress.

Homoeopathy

Homoeopathy is an example of a complete alternative medical system. It was rediscovered in the late 18th century by the German physician Samuel Hahnemann, but is believed to go back even further to the 5th century BC and Hippocrates, the Greek father of medicine. The key principle on which homoeopathic medicine is based is the law of similars or 'like cures like'. According to this law, the same substance that, in large doses, produces the symptoms of a disease will actually cure them if administered in minute doses. Homoeopathic doctors believe that the more diluted a remedy, the more powerful or potent it is. For this reason, they use infinitesimal

HOMEOPATHIC REMEDIES FOR PMS

Suggested remedy	Symptoms
Pulsatilla	Painful breasts
	Tearfulness
	Irregular periods
	Nausea
Sepia	Chilly
	Depressed and weepy
	Low libido
	Tendency to turn on loved ones
	Screaming fits and violence
Nat mur	Irritability or anxiety
	Sadness
	Fluid retention
	Swollen breasts
	Feelings of detachment with headache
	Indifference
Kali mur	Irritability
	Panic attacks
	Anger and tension
	Cravings for sweets and sugar
	Low libido

doses of specially prepared animal, vegetable and mineral sources to stimulate the body's own self-healing mechanism into action.

It's not entirely clear how this works, but homoeopaths believe that the vibrational energy of the remedy stimulates healing by triggering what Hahnemann called the Vital Force, a healing power or energy similar to the Chinese concept of *chi* (see page 91).

For a condition like PMS, the homoeopath may want to prescribe what is known as a constitutional remedy. He or she takes full details of your symptoms, illnesses that run in your family, previous illnesses you have suffered, your likes and dislikes and so on, and prescribes a remedy for you as a whole person. Symptoms will clear in reverse order of their appearance and from the inside outwards, from major to minor organs. You may need different remedies as your symptoms clear. At first there may be an aggravation of symptoms. This is a good sign because it is said to show that the body's self-healing mechanism is kicking into action.

Massage

Tense muscles, caused by emotional tension or physical pain or discomfort, can cause the circulation to become sluggish by forcing the blood vessels to constrict. Massage involves manipulating the body's soft tissues to release emotional tension, relax the muscles and restore blood flow. There are many different kinds of massage. They include sports massage (used to treat sports injury and muscle strain), shiatsu, reflexology, aromatherapy, Indian head massage and bodywork (Thai massage).

The basic techniques are similar in all the different types of massage. They include stroking, kneading, wringing, pummelling and knuckling. Depending on the techniques used, a massage may be energizing or relaxing. Massage can be tremendously helpful for emotional symptoms of PMS, such as anxiety and tension, depression and mood swings. It can also help alleviate fluid retention by stimulating the circulation and lymphatic system.

Reflexology (zone therapy)

Reflexology is a type of massage that consists of applying pressure to reflex points – and sometimes the hands – to stimulate the body's own self-healing mechanism. Therapists claim that applying pressure to these points can improve both mental and physical health.

No one knows exactly how reflexology works but, like acupuncture, it could have something to do with stimulating chemical messengers via the nervous system. Both the hands and the feet are rich in nerve endings.

According to reflexologists, each part of the body has a corresponding point on the feet. So pressing on the part of the feet that corresponds, say, to the endocrine glands or the ovaries, uterus and Fallopian tubes might bring about an improvement in PMS. Although no studies have been done specifically on PMS, one study of reflexology during pregnancy seems to support the idea that it might be of value. In the study, carried out in 1995, 37 pregnant women had a course of reflexology. The group reported shorter, less painful labours than normal, and fewer Caesarean sections. Given that many of the same hormones and hormonal pathways are involved in labour and PMS, it is not too far fetched to think that reflexology may help some of the symptoms of PMS.

Further complementary therapies that may help in PMS

Bach Flower Remedies

Remedies are aimed at helping to ease emotional symptoms. Aspen for anxiety, gorse for depression, crab apple for feelings of self-disgust, cherry plum for feelings of being out of control, mustard for sudden depression, scleranthus for mood swings, and olive and hornbeam for fatigue and tiredness. These herbal remedies are available in health food stores.

Colour therapy

Certain colours are known to affect mood. For example, blue is calming, while red is stimulating and can increase energy. You can use this knowledge in the clothes you choose or the way you decorate your home.

Hypnotherapy

Hypnotherapy is thought to work on the autonomic nervous system which, as we've seen, plays a part in PMS. It's also well established as a treatment for irritable bowel syndrome (IBS).

Naturopathy

Naturopathy involves using elements of nature, such as the food we eat, the air we breathe, water (hydrotherapy) and exercise, to stimulate the body to heal itself. Many of its principles are similar to the lifestyle modifications outlined elsewhere in this book.

6 The role of food in PMS

One of the most important, and enjoyable, things you can do to free yourself from PMS is to eat a healthy diet. Many experts believe that the typical refined Western diet – with its high levels of sugar, salt, alcohol, caffeine and animal fat – is a key factor in the growing numbers of women suffering from PMS, as well as in the rising incidence of heart disease, diabetes, cancer and other degenerative diseases.

In this chapter you will learn about the dietary changes you can make that can, in some cases, cure and in others substantially reduce the symptoms of PMS. The good news is that improving your diet isn't about depriving yourself or restricting what you eat, but about choosing a wide variety of delicious, nutritious food. Once you start eating like this, you'll find you feel so full of zest that you'll want to continue.

Ingredients of a healthy diet

At the end of a busy day, it's easy to grab a ready meal from the freezer or open a packet meal instead of preparing something fresh. There is nothing wrong with this occasionally, but if you do it too often you could be depriving your body of essential nutrients and contributing to your PMS symptoms. In one of the earliest studies on how diet affects PMS, sufferers were found to consume:

- ❑ 62 per cent more refined carbohydrates.
- ❑ 75 per cent more refined sugar.
- ❑ 79 per cent more dairy produce.
- ❑ 78 per cent more salty foods.
- ❑ 53 per cent less iron.
- ❑ 77 per cent less manganese.
- ❑ 52 per cent less zinc than healthy women in the control group.

Experts agree that the best diet for overall good health – and for PMS – is one based around starchy carbohydrate foods, with plenty of fresh fruit and vegetables. It contains a little protein, some dairy (or calcium-containing) foods and a certain amount of unsaturated fats found in vegetables, seeds, nuts and grains, rather than the hard saturated fat found in meat and animal products. Fatty, sugary foods like cakes, biscuits and pastries are best avoided or kept for an occasional treat.

Nutrients such as vitamins, minerals and essential fats work synergistically in the body – that is, they need each other for maximum absorption. A healthy diet above all is a balanced diet. If you eat a variety of fresh foods – all the time, not just when you have PMS – you go a long way towards improving your overall health and gaining control over your symptoms.

The foods you choose to eat should be in as close to their natural state as possible, that is, unprocessed and raw or only lightly cooked.

Diet in detail

Starchy foods

When you have a meal, the biggest portion on your plate should consist of starchy, carbohydrate foods. These include:

❑ Wholegrain cereals, such as brown rice.

❑ Wholegrain pasta.

❑ Couscous.

❑ Breads, such as chapattis and other wholegrain flat breads.

❑ Rye bread.

❑ Starchy vegetables, such as potatoes, yams and sweet potatoes.

Scientists have found that a diet rich in these kinds of foods increases production of the brain chemical serotonin, low levels of which may lie at the root of some of the symptoms of PMS. Starchy foods are also a valuable source of fibre, which can help keep levels of blood sugar balanced, and ease symptoms such as constipation and irritable bowel syndrome, which is often exacerbated by PMS.

Fruit, vegetables, nuts and pulses

Plant-based foods such as salads, pulses, nuts and seeds should be the next biggest portion on your plate. Aim to eat at least five – and preferably more – portions of fruit and vegetables a day. These foods will increase your intake of fibre and of vitamins, minerals and other nutrients, shortages of which may be a key factor in PMS. Fruit and vegetables are also rich in phytochemicals, plant chemicals which help to balance levels of oestrogen and may protect against heart disease, osteoporosis and breast cancer after the menopause.

Vitamins and minerals

The case for calcium Research has shown that many women don't consume enough calcium, especially if they are dieting or restricting their food intake for any reason. Some experts surmise that women with PMS have a calcium deficiency that only comes to light during the second part of their menstrual cycle as hormone levels fluctuate, causing mood swings, irritability and depression. Making sure you get plenty of calcium-rich foods in your diet is, of course, not only a sensible step for helping ease PMS, but will also help build strong bones to protect you against osteoporosis.

Calcium is found in dairy foods. If you don't like or can't eat dairy foods, it's also found in bread, muesli, soya flour, brazil nuts, almonds, sardines, prawns, sprats and whitebait and some brands of bottled water.

The magic of magnesium As we saw on page 71, magnesium is one of the most important nutrients for women with PMS. Magnesium also enhances the absorption of calcium from food, so it's essential if you are to benefit from increasing your intake of calcium. Eating a highly refined diet can leave you short of magnesium. Alcohol, too, can leach magnesium from the body.

Magnesium is found in green leafy vegetables, wholegrain flour, bread, cereals and pasta, peanuts, soya flour, almonds and brazil nuts.

Zinc for zest Zinc is another mineral in which women with PMS may be deficient. It is vital for insulin formation and is important, too, for brain function and the health of the reproductive organs. When taken with vitamin A it can help alleviate premenstrual acne (see page 72). A high caffeine or alcohol level may interfere with the body's absorption of zinc, and you also need more if you are taking large amounts of vitamin B6.

Zinc is found in steak, lamb chops, pork loin, wheatgerm, brewer's yeast, pumpkin seeds, almonds, peanuts, eggs, turkey, muesli and mustard.

Vitamin E Vitamin E is an antioxidant. It can help alleviate fatigue and works as a diuretic and there is evidence that it can help with breast swelling and tenderness.

Vitamin E is found in wheatgerm, soya, broccoli, leafy greens, spinach, whole wheat, wholegrain cereals, hazelnuts, almonds, sunflower oil and eggs.

Chromium counts A shortage of the mineral chromium may be particularly important for protecting against low energy and mood swings caused by dips in blood sugar, as it works with insulin in the metabolism of sugar.

Chromium is found in meat, calves' liver, chicken, shellfish, lamb chops, corn oil, clams and brewer's yeast.

Fats

A high-fat diet can exacerbate the symptoms of PMS, as well, of course, as boosting your risk of obesity, heart disease and other medical problems. Having said that, not all fats are the same.

Certainly the hard saturated fats found in red meat and animal products, such as cheese and sausages, are best kept to a minimum. It's also important to steer clear of transfats – manufactured fats used in bought biscuits, cakes and pastries.

However, certain fats are vital for optimum health. These are the essential fatty acids (EFAs), needed by every cell of our bodies to build healthy cell membranes. EFAs are also used by our bodies to manufacture prostaglandins. These are hormone-like messenger chemicals which are involved in many bodily processes, including control of inflammation, fluid balance, regulation of blood sugar and mental function. Our bodies are not able to manufacture EFAs, so they have to be obtained from food.

There are two kinds of EFAs. Omega-6 is found in nuts, seeds and plant-based foods, evening primrose oil, blackcurrant seed oil and borage oil. Omega-3 is found primarily in oily fish, but also in certain seed oils.

Omega-6 oils have many beneficial effects, but of particular relevance to PMS sufferers is the fact that they are used by the

Sources of Omega-6	Sources of Omega-3
Corn (maize)	Hemp
Hemp	Linseeds
Pumpkin	Pumpkin
Sesame	Herring
Soya	Salmon
Sunflower seeds	Sardines
Walnuts	Swordfish
Wheatgerm	Tuna
Almonds	Mackerel
	Beans
	Spinach
	Wheat

body to make gamma-linoleic acid (GLA), which helps reduce inflammation and pain. This makes them especially useful in treating premenstrual breast tenderness. They may also be helpful in alleviating abdominal cramps. Another property of omega-6 fatty acids is that they help regulate insulin in the blood, so avoiding low blood sugar which can be a cause of tiredness and low mood.

Omega-3 oils are also important for women who suffer from PMS. They are vital for brain function, which in turn can affect concentration and memory, coordination and mood. They are also involved in metabolism, reducing inflammation and maintaining water balance.

Too many animal fats, alcohol, infections and deficiencies of other vitamins and minerals can all reduce your body's ability to metabolize essential fatty acids.

Note: See page 66 for more information on essential fatty acids and GLA. If you have a blood disorder or bleeding problems, fish oils should only be taken after you have sought the advice of your doctor.

Increasing your intake of essential fatty acids

❑ The first step in ensuring you get a good supply of omega-6 and omega-3 EFAs is to make sure that you are eating a healthy nutritious diet.

❑ Watch your cooking methods. Avoid frying, apart from brief stir-frying using a seed oil such as sesame.

❑ Cut down on animal fats.

❑ Eat plenty of vegetables, salads, nuts and seeds.

❑ Avoid alcohol and smoking.

❑ Avoid refined carbohydrates.

- Make up a seed mix and use it to sprinkle on cereals or salads. Dry-toasting them briefly in a nonstick frying pan gives them a fabulous crunchy texture.
- Consider taking a supplement.
- Omega-6 and omega-3 work in harmony, so you must get both (see above).
- EFAs need magnesium, vitamin C, zinc and vitamins B3 and B6 to work effectively. Make sure you get a plentiful supply, either through your diet or by taking a multivitamin and mineral supplement.

Organic foods

Another measure that may improve symptoms of PMS is to go organic. Environmental oestrogens – known as xenoestrogens, literally 'foreign oestrogens' – are found in certain pesticides used to spray fruit and vegetables and in additives used in meat. They are thought to disrupt the body's production of natural oestrogen by latching on to oestrogen receptors. They are also believed to meddle with the way the body's sex hormones work. Switching to a vegetarian diet, or at least putting more vegetarian dishes on the menu, and buying organic meat, fruit and vegetable whenever you can, will help reduce your exposure to these compounds and reduce your intake of animal fat, which is where xenoestrogens are stored.

Water

Drinking plenty of water will help you absorb nutrients from food, aid weight loss if you are overweight and help maintain your body's fluid balance. Contrary to popular perception, restricting what you drink actually aggravates rather than alleviates bloating. Caffeinated drinks can contribute to bloating too, so stick to plain water or herbal teas. Aim to drink at least eight glasses a day (about 2.5 litres/4 pints), or more when you are exercising.

Foods to avoid

While eating to alleviate PMS is mostly about things you can eat and drink, there are a few foods and beverages you should avoid. Some of these are best avoided altogether, or eaten only in limited quantities, by anyone who wants to eat more healthily. Others are mentioned because they may trigger symptoms in PMS sufferers – a certain degree of trial and error may be necessary to see if this is true for you.

Sugar

Sugar is present in sweets, biscuits and pastries, and is also a hidden ingredient in many processed foods like breakfast cereals and even savoury foods and snacks. Many women with PMS seem to be especially sensitive to the effects of sugar, which can cause a rise in insulin. This can in turn lead to fluid retention and also increase the excretion of magnesium.

Wheat

Wholegrain cereals are, as we have seen, the mainstay of a healthy diet. However, some women with PMS may be sensitive to wheat or to gluten, a type of protein found in wheat and other grains. If this applies to you, avoiding wheat can sometimes bring dramatic relief in symptoms, especially where bloating and irritable bowel syndrome (IBS) are causing problems.

Salt

Most of us consume far too much salt (sodium). Even if you don't use salt in cooking or sprinkle it on your food, if you eat a highly refined diet you will be consuming hidden salt in processed foods. Too much salt is associated with a risk of high blood pressure, heart disease and also boosts the risk of osteoporosis and stomach cancer.

More to the point, it can aggravate bloating, breast tenderness and water retention. And while the fluid retention of PMS is primarily caused by hormone-linked changes in the body's fluid balance, a high intake of salt can certainly make matters worse. Research shows that lowering your salt intake can lead to an instant weight loss of up to five pounds (2.3 kg). To do this, avoid processed foods and don't add salt to food in cooking or at the table.

Incidentally, fruit and vegetables are rich in potassium, which helps control the body's sodium balance – yet another good reason to increase your intake of these foods.

Red meat

There is evidence to suggest that women eating a diet containing a lot of red meat are more prone to PMS. Although red meat is high in iron, an essential nutrient for women of reproductive age, it is also rich in saturated fats, which can, as we've seen, block the formation of prostaglandins. Red meat can also aggravate symptoms of IBS. It may be worth cutting out red meat altogether for a time to see if this helps. Instead of red meat, eat fish, poultry and game, which are low in saturated fats, and whole grains and dark green vegetables to make sure you're getting enough iron.

Caffeine

Caffeine, found in coffee, tea, cola and other caffeinated soft drinks, is a stimulant. Although it may give you a temporary lift, it can actually worsen symptoms of anxiety, irritability, headaches and migraine. Too much caffeine can also aggravate breast tenderness and has a powerful effect on the bowel, which can worsen symptoms of premenstrual IBS.

Caffeine competes with natural chemicals in the brain and alters the natural flow of your body's own feel-good hormones. If you have mild to moderate PMS, try cutting down your caffeine intake to a couple of cups of tea a day and one cup of coffee. For more severe symptoms, it's worth cutting out caffeine altogether and sticking to water, decaffeinated coffees and herbal teas. It's best to wean yourself off caffeine in the early part of your menstrual cycle, as you may initially experience withdrawal symptoms such as nervousness, shakiness and headaches, which will be harder to deal with before your period.

Alcohol

A moderate intake of alcohol can be part of a healthy diet. However, in excess it can worsen PMS. Some women crave alcohol before their periods, but there's evidence that PMS sufferers may be more sensitive to its effects. Alcohol, like refined sugar, causes a swift rise followed by a drop in blood sugar. It is also a depressant, can interfere with sleep patterns and irritate the bowel.

If your PMS is mild to moderate, you may be able to tolerate a couple of small glasses of wine a day (fewer than 14 units a week). If you suffer severe PMS, however, it may be worth cutting out alcohol completely for a while to see if your symptoms subside. If you do drink alcohol, always make sure you eat something at the same time as drinking on an empty stomach increases its effects.

Food sensitivity?

Although some conventional doctors dismiss the idea, many nutritional experts believe that food allergy or intolerance may be a factor in causing PMS or making it worse. Food allergy in its strict sense involves an immune reaction that happens immediately after eating a specific food. Far more common is food intolerance, or delayed sensitivity, to a food.

Keeping a diary of what you eat and your symptoms can help identify if food sensitivity is a factor in causing your PMS. If it is, you may find your symptoms are much better if you eliminate the offending food or foods. Having said this, leaving foods out of your diet can leave you at risk of deficiencies of essential nutrients – something that should be avoided at all costs if you have PMS. If you do leave something out of your diet, make sure you substitute another source of the nutrients it contains. If this proves difficult, seek the advice of your doctor or dietician.

Moderating your diet
Foods to choose

❏ Fresh fruit and vegetables, preferably organic.
❏ Chicken, fish and game, preferably organic.
❏ Wholegrain cereals and starchy vegetables.
❏ Nuts, seeds and their oils.
❏ Herbal teas, decaffeinated coffees and water.

Foods to avoid

❑ Processed and fast foods.

❑ Red meat.

❑ Biscuits, cakes and pastries made with refined sugar and white flour.

❑ Hard saturated fats found in sausages, pies and patisserie.

❑ Coffee, tea, drinking chocolate, cola, soft drinks and alcohol.

Food cravings – what your body is trying to tell you

Shortages of nutrients can, as we have seen, be an important contributory factor in PMS, while calorific requirements can climb by up to 500 calories per day in the second half of your menstrual cycle. This is especially true if you are restricting your diet, either because you're watching your weight or because you're cutting out certain foods for other reasons. Many experts believe that food cravings are the body's way of trying to meet its needs – both for nutrients and for extra calories. It's wise to listen to your body and if you're on a weight-loss diet to ease up premenstrually. This doesn't mean wolfing down a load of fatty, sugary foods, but do try to make sure that you get three good meals and a couple of wholesome snacks each day. You'll probably find that you want to eat more lightly once you actually start your period, and that your calorie count balances out over the course of the month.

Patterns of eating

How you eat is every bit as important as what you eat in controlling symptoms of PMS. Eating little and often will ensure that you get all the nutrients you need, while eliminating fluctuations in blood sugar which may contribute to symptoms. Conversely, skipping meals, eating on the run or when you are feeling stressed can exacerbate them. When you eat make sure it is in a peaceful, stress-free environment and that you are relaxed. If you know you have a busy day ahead, pack a substantial salad or a flask of soup for your lunch (see Chapter 7 for ideas) and a couple of healthy snacks to get you through the day.

Starting to eat more healthily

If you lead a busy life, it can be hard to change your eating habits and start eating more healthily. Shopping for and cooking fresh ingredients can be more time-consuming than reaching for a packet or a ready meal. However, it's also more

---

SNACK ATTACK

Eat unrefined, natural foods as snacks and avoid fatty, sugary foods. Try any of the following:

○ Puffed grains, such as air-popped popcorn.
○ Fruit – fresh, dried or cooked. Combine these with a low to moderate glycaemic index (see page 118).
○ Wholegrain rye bread or soda bread with a sugar-free preserve or mashed banana.
○ Rice cakes.
○ Seeds and nuts, such as pumpkin, sunflower, almonds, hazelnuts, pecans.
○ Yogurt and fruit.

---

satisfying to eat a meal that you have prepared yourself, that you know contains only the freshest and most nutritious ingredients – and the bonus, both in terms of increased health and vitality and the abating of your PMS, will more than repay your efforts.

At the end of this chapter (pages 122–123) you'll find some sample menu plans that will help to make it easier. And in Chapter 7 you'll discover a host of inspiring recipes from which to choose.

If you are starting to make healthy food choices for the first time, congratulate yourself. Changing your habits takes courage and determination, and it isn't something that happens overnight. It can take up to three or four months to see the benefits of a changed diet, so be patient and don't be too hard on yourself if you have the occasional lapse.

Top tips for success

Be prepared Many of us rush into making changes in health habits before we're really ready. Slow down and first make a list of everything you will gain from eating more healthily.

Picture this Rather than focusing on how lousy you feel now, imagine how much healthier you'll be if you eat a nutritious diet. Imagine how you'll feel – and look – in six months, a year, five years.

Get information Check out books, articles, the Internet, your doctor, friends and relatives for ideas. Focus on the positive aspects of healthy eating – the tasty foods you can eat rather than those you can't.

Find your motivator We all approach things differently, so think about the way to change your eating habits that best suits you: some people like to make changes gradually, while others prefer a clean sweep. It doesn't matter which route you go so long as you feel happy.

Clean up your kitchen Clear your fridge and cupboards of unhealthy food, and stock up on fresh fruit and vegetables, popcorn, rice cakes and other healthy snacks.

Forgive your lapses Half of people lapse within three months of making any major health change such as eating a healthy diet, stopping smoking or cutting down on drinking. This doesn't mean you have to abandon your healthy eating plan. The secret of permanent change is to accept your lapse – and carry on.

Plan for lapses Not sticking to good resolutions is demoralizing. But attributing your lapse to lack of willpower or what a terrible person you are is even more damaging. Most women who lapse when they are premenstrual do so because they are busy, depressed, tired or anxious. Ask yourself, 'How am I going to deal with it next time around?'

Do it for a month and see how you feel It's easier to commit to something for a short time and it proves that you can do it. After a month you'll probably feel healthier, more energetic and more in control. Use these feelings to encourage yourself to stick to the changes you've made for another month, another, and then another.

Be patient Changing your diet isn't an instant fix. Bear in mind that it can take up to three or four months to feel the benefits, but by the end of that time you should have begun to feel significantly better physically and mentally.

Food and physical symptoms of PMS

Many of the physical symptoms of PMS, like acne and rashes, changed bowel habits, headaches, bloating and breast tenderness, can be affected by what you eat. Following the healthy diet rules previously outlined will help. The chart overleaf sums up all the dietary measures to try.

Food and mood

What you eat and drink can have a significant effect on the emotional and mental symptoms of PMS. In the past few years, there has been an avalanche of studies into how food effects mood, fuelled by the discovery that certain nutrients can affect the behaviour of brain chemicals.

There is growing evidence, for example, that the balance of protein and carbohydrate in meals can affect levels of serotonin which, as we've seen, is linked to symptoms such as lowered mood and food cravings.

Low mood, anxiety, fatigue and lack of energy have been associated with imbalances in a number of nutrients. They include calcium, vitamin D, magnesium, zinc, chromium, vitamin E, the B vitamins and essential fatty acids.

It will be several years before experts unravel the full picture on exactly how food affects mood before a period. However, there are some tantalizing clues that can help you begin to manage your PMS more effectively right now.

Symptom	Potential causes
Acne and spots	Increased sensitivity to hormonal changes in the skin. Zinc deficiency.
Bloating	Changes in the body's fluid balance induced by hormonal changes.
Constipation	Sluggish movements of the bowel caused by the action of progesterone on the smooth muscle tissue of the bowel.
Breast tenderness	Can be linked with smoking and caffeine found in tea, coffee, soft drinks and 'alcopops'. Also linked with foods rich in animal fats, and transfatty acids found in pastries, cakes and biscuits.
Irritable bowel syndrome	Menstrual magnification of existing problems.
Headaches and migraine	Lowered threshold, possibly caused by lowered blood sugar resulting from hormonal changes, food sensitivities, stress and tension. Dietary triggers, e.g. cheese, chocolate, coffee, monosodium glutamate, oranges, shellfish, yeast and meat extracts, smoked and pickled fish, red wine.
Weight gain (caused by food cravings)	Low blood sugar levels, possibly caused by lack of chromium, magnesium, vitamins B and C, and exacerbated by tension and stress.

Dietary steps

- ○ Eat a healthy diet.
- ○ Oily fish may help.
- ○ Drink plenty of water.
- ○ Multivitamin supplement.
- ○ Zinc supplement.

- ○ Eat a healthy diet.
- ○ Cut out salt.
- ○ Avoid processed foods.
- ○ Avoid fatty, sugary foods.
- ○ Step up consumption of essential fatty acids.

- ○ Eat a healthy diet.
- ○ Pay particular attention to fruit and vegetables and other high-fibre foods.
- ○ Sprinkle linseed over breakfast cereal.

- ○ Eat a healthy diet.
- ○ Avoid butter, margarine, cakes, pastries and biscuits.
- ○ Cut down on salt.
- ○ Restrict dairy products.
- ○ Avoid caffeine.
- ○ Increase magnesium consumption.
- ○ Increase essential fatty acids.
- ○ Evening primrose oil supplement.

- ○ Eat a healthy high-fibre diet.
- ○ Check for food sensitivities, e.g. wheat, dairy products.
- ○ Avoid coffee, alcohol and spicy foods.

- ○ Eat a healthy diet.
- ○ Eat little and often.
- ○ Avoid sugar.
- ○ Avoid tea, coffee and chocolate.
- ○ Check for dietary triggers and avoid if applicable.

- ○ Eat a healthy diet.
- ○ Eat little and often.
- ○ Relax and enjoy your meals.
- ○ Choose naturally sweet foods like dried fruit, fresh fruit, nuts and seeds, rather than sweets and bought biscuits.
- ○ Take a supplement of vitamin B, magnesium and chromium to correct blood sugar levels.

Sustaining energy levels

Low energy and fatigue, as we've seen, is one of the most common symptoms of PMS. Eating a healthy diet can do much to keep your energy levels on a more even keel and eliminate dips in blood sugar, which can play havoc with your mood, especially premenstrually.

Your brain plays an important part in PMS and one thing it needs is a constant supply of blood sugar or glucose. Whenever you eat, glucose levels in your blood rise, dropping over the next few hours until you have your next meal. If you skip meals or restrict what you eat, you are setting yourself up for a low blood sugar level, which can lead to fatigue, irritability and depression – symptoms that are all too well known to anyone with PMS.

Everything you eat is broken down and used by your body to supply energy: fats are stored to provide long-term energy, proteins are used for muscle building and repair and sugars and starchy foods are used to supply instant energy. Sugars and starches are broken down during digestion into glucose. Any spare glucose is converted into a compound called glycogen, which is stored in your liver and muscles. When your body needs energy, these glycogen stores are mobilized to give you an instant shot.

The glycaemic index

The glycaemic index (GI) is a measure of how rapidly your body breaks down starchy and sugary foods, and the speed with which sugar levels in the blood rise after eating the food.

Some foods – in particular refined starchy and sugary foods like cakes, biscuits, sweets and soft drinks – have what is known as a high glycaemic index. They cause blood sugar levels to soar soon after eating them, giving you an instant burst of energy. Unfortunately, a high blood sugar level triggers the release of the hormone insulin from the pancreas, which soon causes the level to plummet again, leaving you feeling tired, irritable and hungry. A number of healthy carbohydrates, such as bread, rice, corn, potatoes, cooked carrots and bananas, also provide a similar quick-fix of blood sugar.

If you want to maintain even levels of energy, you are better off opting for healthy foods with a low or moderate GI that raise blood sugar levels more slowly. Low-GI foods also increase production of the brain chemical serotonin, which helps control appetite as well as improving mood.

There is evidence that women with PMS have falling blood sugar levels, which could be another reason why so many women crave sugary, starchy foods premenstrually. Unfortunately, if you attempt to fix this problem by eating foods with a high GI, you may find that all you do is exacerbate the problem.

The glycaemic index of some common foods

High Baked potato, bananas, bought biscuits, broad beans, brown rice, cooked carrots, cornflakes, crackers, glucose honey, mashed potato, muesli, parsnip, popcorn, raisins, soft drinks, sweetcorn, watermelon, wheat-based cereals, white rice, white bread, wholegrain bread.

Moderate Beetroot, 'healthier' biscuits, boiled potatoes, bran-based cereals, brown bread, chocolate bar, corn (maize) crisps, frozen peas, grapes, new potatoes, noodles, oatmeal biscuits, oats, oranges, pineapple, pitta bread, porridge, refined breakfast cereals with sugar, sponge cake, sweet potatoes, white pasta, wholemeal pasta, yam.

Low Apples, apricots, baked beans, beetroot, butter beans, cherries, chickpeas, dark chocolate, fresh peas, fructose (or fruit sugar), grapefruit, green vegetables, ice cream, kidney beans, lemon, lentils, lima beans, milk, mushrooms, peaches, plums, peanuts, skimmed milk, soya beans, soya milk, sugar-free fruit preserves, tomatoes, wholegrain rye bread, whole milk, yogurt.

DO YOU NEED A SUPPLEMENT?

Ideally, eating a healthy diet should supply all the vitamins and minerals you need. Unfortunately, with the busy lives most of us lead today, we don't always eat as well as we should. Futhermore, environmental factors such as pollution, factory farming, the use of pesticides and food additives, and aspects of modern living, such as increased stress levels, smoking, drinking alcohol and the contraceptive pill, can rob the body of nutrients making women vulnerable to PMS.

If the dietary measures in this chapter don't banish your PMS, you may find a supplement is beneficial (see pages 68–72). However, bear in mind that supplements are just that – an addition to a healthy, nutritious diet, not a substitute. In order for them to work, you should also be eating a well-balanced diet.

B vitamins and energy

There is sometimes an association between fatigue and a deficiency of one of the B-complex vitamins. B-complex vitamins include thiamin (B1), riboflavin (B2), niacin, vitamin B6 (pyridoxine), B12, biotin, pantothenic acid and folic acid. Thiamin, riboflavin and niacin are vital for the release of energy from carbohydrates or fats. Because they are soluble in water, B vitamins are not stored in the body. Even a mild shortage of these vitamins can affect your energy levels. B vitamins are found in wholegrain cereals, nuts, seeds, pulses, eggs, green leafy vegetables, sprouted seeds, rye and many other foods.

Maintaining energy

❑ Try to include one or more low-GI foods with each meal.
❑ Never skip breakfast. Scientific research has confirmed the truth of the saying, 'Breakfast like a king, lunch like a prince and dine like a pauper'.
❑ Aim to combine foods with a low and high GI, for example a bowl of cornflakes with a chopped peach or plum, mashed banana on a slice of rye bread, a bowl of muesli topped with yogurt and a handful of cherries.
❑ Eat little and often – eating a small snack between breakfast and lunch, and lunch and supper, will help keep energy levels topped up.
❑ Combining protein with carbohydrate can be beneficial. So, for example, have a poached egg on wholemeal toast, pesto and pasta or hummus with pitta bread.
❑ Include foods high in B vitamins at every meal.
❑ Consider taking a B-complex vitamin supplement.

Menu suggestions

MILD TO MODERATE PMS

Meal	Foods
Breakfast	○ Warm honey and raisin muffins (see page 133) ○ Herbal tea or decaffeinated coffee
Snack	○ Mashed banana on a slice of wholegrain rye bread or rice cake ○ Herbal tea
Lunch	○ Salade niçoise (see page 150) ○ Wholemeal bread ○ Fruit juice
Snack	○ Date and walnut bread (see page 220) ○ Herbal tea with a slice of ginger
Supper	○ Fruit and nut couscous and chicken skewers (see page 196) ○ Steamed courgettes, carrots and red peppers ○ Fig and honey pots (see page 217) ○ Still mineral water
Before bed	○ Camomile or lemon balm tea ○ Dry-popped popcorn

How they help

Dried fruits are rich in potassium, which helps control fluid balance in the body, and iron, which helps combat anaemia. They also contain fructose (fruit sugar), which has a low GI index and helps maintain energy levels.

Banana has a high glycaemic index and will help give you a rapid energy boost, as well as potassium. Combined with wholegrain rye bread, which has a low glycaemic index, it will help maintain sustained energy levels. Banana is also a source of magnesium, which is often lacking in women with PMS.

Oily fish, such as tuna, is rich in omega-3 fatty acids. Fresh tuna is low in salt, which helps to reduce swelling and bloating. Leave out the seasoning if you suffer from bloating. Wholemeal bread will help ease constipation and help to maintain energy levels. It's also a good source of chromium. Fruit juice is a rich source of vitamin C, which helps the absorption of iron.

Calorie needs are higher during the premenstrual period. A wholesome snack will help sustain you, making you less likely to reach for the biscuit tin. Wholemeal flour is a source of B vitamins and fibre. Walnuts are rich in beneficial essential fatty acids and vitamin B. Dates contain iron and are rich in B vitamins. Ginger contains anti-inflammatory chemicals that help quell headaches and migraine.

Chicken is low in fat and high in protein, and is also a source of vitamin E. Dried fruits contain potassium, which helps balance fluid levels. The natural yogurt in the fig and honey pots provides calcium and probiotic bacteria, which help maintain balanced levels of bacteria in the gut. Red peppers and carrots are a good source of magnesium, as well as beta-carotene (one of the antioxidant vitamins). Figs are rich in soluble fibre, which helps ease IBS symptoms, as well as potassium, calcium and iron. Mineral water is a good source of calcium.

Popcorn is low in fat and will help keep energy levels stable while you sleep. Camomile and lemon balm are calming.

SEVERE PMS

Meal	Foods
Breakfast	○ Granola (see page 128) with sliced bananas and natural yogurt ○ Herbal tea or decaffeinated coffee
Snack	○ Date and walnut bread (see page 220) ○ Herbal tea or decaffeinated coffee
Lunch	○ Jacket potato with tuna in spring water ○ Celery, red onion and new potato salad (see page 144) ○ Fruit juice
Snack	○ Piece of fresh fruit ○ Camomile tea ○ Bowl of dry-popped popcorn
Supper	○ Roasted pepper soup (see page 136) ○ Grilled chicken sala thai style (see page 198) ○ Fresh fruit salad sprinkled with chopped hazelnuts ○ Lemon grass tea
Before bed	○ Camomile tea ○ Rice cakes

How they help

A sustaining breakfast will set you up for the day and help avoid dips in blood sugar, which can lead to tiredness, mood swings and low energy. This granola is high in unrefined carbohydrates and soluble fibre. It also contains B vitamins for the nerves, vitamin E, vitamin C and potassium to help regulate fluid balance. Bananas are a source of chromium, which helps break down sugar, and potassium to balance fluid levels.

This high-carbohydrate snack will help sustain you and is low in fat and sugar. Walnuts are a good source of essential fatty acids and dates and molasses are rich in iron.

Jacket potatoes and the vegetables in this salad contain soluble dietary fibre, which helps regulate the bowels. Celery contains potassium which helps balance fluid levels in the body.

Fruit is generally well tolerated and helps ease bloating. Camomile tea is calming.

A low-fat, high-protein, vitamin- and mineral-rich dish. Ginger is an anti-inflammatory which helps ease headaches and migraine, and also contains vitamin B2. Sesame seeds are a good source of calcium. Hot red chillies are a good source of vitamin B2. Fresh fruit is rich in vitamin C and hazelnuts are a good source of magnesium. Leave out the red food colouring and substitute apple juice for wine if you have food sensitivities.

Rice cakes will help prevent dips in blood sugar while you sleep. Camomile will help calm and relax you.

7 Recipes to beat PMS

This section contains a selection of tasty, well-balanced recipes, chosen to help banish the symptoms of PMS. There is a strong emphasis on whole foods and fruit and vegetables, ensuring you get all the nutrients you need – especially calcium, magnesium, zinc, chromium, B vitamins and essential fatty acids, which have been shown to be important in preventing PMS.

If you're watching your salt intake, feel free to adapt and experiment with other seasonings like garlic, fresh herbs, spices and ginger. Also, if food sensitivity might be a factor, you can substitute other ingredients for any that cause you problems.

It is vital to eat little and often to prevent food cravings, keep up nutrient levels and prevent dips in blood sugar. Above all, eating to beat PMS is about learning just how delicious healthy, nutritious food can be.

Breakfasts

Granola

alcohol free ✓ | citrus free ✓ | dairy free ✓ | gluten free ✗ | wheat free ✓

Serves 18 (3 heaped tablespoons per portion)
Preparation time: 10 minutes, plus cooling
Cooking time: 20 minutes

Per serving
Energy 220 kcals/923 kJ | Protein 5 g | Carbohydrate 25 g | Fat 12 g
Fibre 3 g

100 ml (3½ fl oz) safflower oil
40 ml (1½ fl oz) malt extract
75 ml (3 fl oz) clear honey
325 g (11 oz) rolled oats
250 g (8 oz) jumbo oats (large oat flakes)
50 g (2 oz) hazelnuts
25 g (1 oz) desiccated coconut
50 g (2 oz) sunflower seeds
25 g (1 oz) sesame seeds

1 Put the oil, malt and honey into a large saucepan and heat gently until the malt is runny. Mix in the remaining ingredients and stir thoroughly.

2 Turn into a large roasting tin and bake in a preheated oven at 190°C (375°F), Gas Mark 5, for about 20 minutes, stirring occasionally, until golden brown. Leave to cool, then separate into pieces with your fingers.

3 Store in an airtight container. Serve with natural yogurt at breakfast time, or use as a topping for fresh fruit salad or stewed fruits.

Potato cakes

alcohol free ✓ I citrus free ✓ I dairy free ✓ I gluten free ✓ I wheat free ✓

Serves 4
Preparation time: 10 minutes
Cooking time: 20 minutes

Per serving
Energy 194 kcal/814 kJ I Protein 9 g I Carbohydrate 25 g I Fat 9 g
Fibre 3 g

500 g (1 lb) potatoes, grated
1 onion, chopped
2 tablespoons chopped parsley
2 eggs, beaten
2 tablespoons olive oil
salt and pepper

1 Put the grated potatoes into a colander and rinse under cold running water to remove excess starch.

2 Put the potatoes into a bowl with the onion, parsley, eggs and salt and pepper to taste. Mix thoroughly.

3 Heat the oil in a 20–23 cm (8–9 inch) heavy-based frying pan. Add the potato mixture and pat lightly into a cake. Fry gently for about 8–10 minutes, until the underside is crisp and brown.

4 Slide the potato cake on to a plate, then invert it back into the pan and fry the other side for 10 minutes, until crisp and brown. Using a cutter, stamp the potato cake into rounds. Alternatively, cut the potato cake into wedges. Season with salt and pepper and serve immediately.

Warm honey and raisin muffins

alcohol free ✓ | citrus free ✓ | dairy free ✗ | gluten free ✗ | wheat free ✗

Makes 12
Preparation time: 15 minutes
Cooking time: 15–20 minutes

Per serving
Energy 126 kcal/529 kJ | Protein 4 g | Carbohydrate 16 g | Fat 5 g
Fibre 1 g

125 g (4 oz) wheatgerm
2 teaspoons baking powder
pinch of salt
75 g (3 oz) raisins
4 tablespoons clear honey
50 g (2 oz) butter or margarine, melted
2 small eggs
about 6 tablespoons milk

1 Put the wheatgerm, baking powder, salt and raisins into a bowl, then add the honey, butter or margarine and eggs. Mix until blended, then stir in enough milk to make a fairly soft mixture, which drops heavily from the spoon when you shake it.

2 Put heaped tablespoons of the mixture into greased muffin tins, dividing the mixture among the 12 sections. Bake in a preheated oven at 180°C (350°F), Gas Mark 4, for 15–20 minutes, until the muffins have puffed up and feel firm to a light touch. Serve warm.

Soups

Gazpacho andaluz

alcohol free ✓ | citrus free ✗ | dairy free ✓ | gluten free ✗ | wheat free ✗

Serves 8
Preparation time: 20 minutes, plus chilling
Cooking time: 5 minutes

Per serving
Energy 87 kcal/370 kJ | Protein 4 g | Carbohydrate 17 g | Fat 1 g
Fibre 3 g

125 g (4 oz) onion, finely diced
125 g (4 oz) green pepper, cored, deseeded and finely diced
125 g (4 oz) red pepper, cored, deseeded and finely diced
375 g (12 oz) cucumber, peeled and finely diced
750 g (1½ lb) well-flavoured red tomatoes, skinned, deseeded and
  coarsely chopped
400 g (13 oz) can chopped plum tomatoes
3 garlic cloves, crushed
3 tablespoons double concentrate tomato purée
500 ml (17 fl oz) tomato juice
150–300 ml (¼–½ pint) water
1½ teaspoons soft brown sugar
1 teaspoon oregano, chopped
5 tablespoons red wine vinegar
salt and pepper
snipped chives, to garnish

Croûtons:
3 slices bread
1½ tablespoons lemon juice

1. Reserve about 4 tablespoons each of the onion, green and red peppers and cucumber for the garnish. Put the remaining diced vegetables into a food processor or blender with the fresh and canned tomatoes, garlic and tomato purée. Blend until smooth.

2. Add the tomato juice, water to taste, sugar, oregano and wine vinegar, then process again until well mixed. Season with salt and pepper. Transfer to a large bowl or measuring jug, cover and chill for at least 2 hours.

3. Meanwhile, make the croûtons. Remove the crusts from 3 slices of bread and brush both sides of the bread with lemon juice. Toast the bread until pale brown on both sides. Cut into cubes or long strips.

4. Just before serving, divide the reserved diced vegetables between 8 chilled soup plates. Pour the cold soup on top. Serve with the croûtons and garnish with chives.

Bean and cabbage soup

alcohol free ✓ | citrus free ✓ | dairy free ✓ | gluten free ✗ | wheat free ✗

Serves 4
Preparation time: 15 minutes, plus soaking
Cooking time about 2¼ hours

Per serving
Energy 420 kcals/1750 kJ | Protein 25 g | Carbohydrate 33 g | Fat 21 g
Fibre 3 g

175 g (6 oz) dried broad beans, soaked overnight in cold water
250 g (8 oz) chorizo sausage for cooking
2 rosemary sprigs
bouquet garni
1.8 litres (3 pints) cold water
2 tablespoons olive oil
1 onion, chopped
2 garlic cloves, crushed
1 small red pepper, cored, deseeded and chopped
pinch of cayenne pepper
250 g (8 oz) Savoy cabbage, shredded
1 tablespoon chopped parsley
salt and pepper

To serve:
olive oil
crusty bread

1 Drain and rinse the soaked beans. Put them into a saucepan with 125 g (4 oz) of the chorizo in a piece, the rosemary, bouquet garni and cold water. Bring to the boil and boil rapidly for 10 minutes, then simmer gently, covered, for 1–1½ hours, until the beans are tender.

2 Heat the oil in a frying pan and fry the onion, garlic, red pepper and cayenne for 5 minutes. Dice the remaining chorizo, add to the pan and fry for a further 5 minutes.

3 Stir the onion mixture into the cooked beans with the cabbage and salt and pepper to taste. Bring to the boil and cook for 20 minutes. Add the parsley, adjust the seasoning and spoon into warmed bowls. Drizzle with olive oil and serve immediately with crusty bread.

Roasted pepper soup with black pepper cream

alcohol free ✓ | citrus free ✓ | dairy free ✗ | gluten free ✗ | wheat free ✗

Serves 4
Preparation time: 20 minutes
Cooking time: 1 hour

Per serving

Energy 219 kcals/909 kJ | Protein 4 g | Carbohydrate 13 g | Fat 17 g
Fibre 5 g

6 large red or yellow peppers

4 leeks, white and pale green parts only, thinly sliced

3 tablespoons olive oil

750 ml (1¼ pints) chicken or vegetable stock

2 teaspoons black peppercorns

75 ml (3 fl oz) mascarpone cheese

75 ml (3 fl oz) milk

salt and pepper

toasted country bread, to serve

1 Put the peppers into a large roasting tin and roast in a preheated oven at 240°C (475°F), Gas Mark 9, for 20–30 minutes, turning once, until they begin to char. Remove the peppers from the oven, put them into a polythene bag and close it tightly. Leave for 10 minutes to steam.

2 Put the leeks into a bowl of cold water to soak for 5 minutes.

3 Remove the peppers from the bag and peel off the skins, then pull out the stalks – the seeds should come with them. Halve the peppers, scrape out any remaining seeds and roughly chop the flesh. Swish the leeks around in the water to loosen any mud, then drain and rinse well.

4 Heat the oil in a large saucepan, add the leeks and cook gently for 10 minutes, until soft but not coloured. Add the peppers, stock and a little salt and pepper. Bring the mixture to the boil, then turn down the heat and simmer for 20 minutes.

5 Pound or grind the black peppercorns as finely as possible. Beat the mascarpone with the milk and pepper. Season with salt and chill until needed.

6 Liquidize the soup in a food processor or blender, then pass it through a sieve back into the rinsed out pan. Reheat, taste and adjust the seasoning if necessary. Serve the soup in warmed bowls with dollops of the pepper cream and slices of toasted country bread.

Pumpkin and garlic soup

alcohol free ✓ | citrus free ✓ | dairy free ✗ | gluten free ✓ | wheat free ✓

Serves 6–8
Preparation time: 30 minutes
Cooking time: 50 minutes

Per serving
Energy 228 kcals/947 kJ | Protein 11 g | Carbohydrate 14 g | Fat 15 g
Fibre 2 g

750 g (1½ lb) pumpkin
6 garlic cloves, unpeeled
4 tablespoons olive oil
2 onions, finely sliced
2 celery sticks, chopped
50 g (2 oz) white long-grain rice
1.5 litres (2½ pints) chicken or vegetable stock, or water
salt and pepper
4 tablespoons chopped parsley, to serve

Parmesan crisps:
125 g (4 oz) freshly grated Parmesan cheese
a few fennel seeds (optional)
fresh red chilli, finely chopped (optional)

1 Scrape out the seeds from the pumpkin, cut off the skin and cut the flesh into large cubes. Put them into a roasting tin with the garlic cloves and toss with 2 tablespoons of the olive oil. Do not crowd the tin – use 2 tins if necessary. Roast in a preheated oven at 200°C (400°F), Gas Mark 6, for about 30 minutes, until the pumpkin is very tender and beginning to brown a little.

2 Heat the remaining olive oil in a large saucepan and add the onions and celery. Cook over a gentle heat for 10 minutes, until they are just beginning to brown and soften. Stir in the rice and pour in the stock or water. Bring to the boil, cover the pan and simmer for about 15–20 minutes, until the rice is tender.

3 Remove the pumpkin and garlic from the oven and let them cool slightly. Then pop the garlic cloves out of their skins. Add the garlic and pumpkin to the saucepan, bring to the boil and simmer for 10 minutes.

4 To make the Parmesan crisps, first line a baking sheet with nonstick baking parchment. Spoon small mounds of cheese onto the paper at regular intervals. Flatten with the back of a spoon. Sprinkle some fennel seeds and chopped chilli on top, if liked.

5 Bake the crisps in a preheated oven at 200°C (400°F), Gas Mark 6, for 3–6 minutes, until golden. Remove from the oven and leave for a couple of minutes to set, or, if you prefer, curl them over a rolling pin or a wooden spoon at this stage. Carefully lift them off the paper. Put to one side and leave to cool completely.

6 Liquidize or blend the soup in a food processor or blender and return it to the pan. Taste and season with salt and freshly ground black pepper. Add extra stock or water if the soup is too thick.

7 To serve, reheat the soup and stir in the parsley. Serve with the Parmesan crisps.

Caldo verde

alcohol free ✓ | citrus free ✕ | dairy free ✓ | gluten free ✕ | wheat free ✕

Serves 6
Preparation time: 10 minutes
Cooking time: 40 minutes

Per serving
Energy 125 kcal/520kJ | Protein 4 g | Carbohydrate 19 g | Fat 4 g
Fibre 5 g

2 tablespoons olive oil
1 large onion, chopped
2 garlic cloves, chopped
500 g (1 lb) potatoes, cut into 2.5 cm (1 inch) cubes
1.2 litres (2 pints) water or vegetable stock
250 g (8 oz) spring greens, finely shredded
2 tablespoons chopped parsley
salt and pepper
croûtons (see page 132), to serve

1 Heat the oil in a large frying pan and fry the onion for 5 minutes, until softened but not brown. Add the garlic and potatoes and cook for a few minutes, stirring occasionally.

2 Add the water or stock, season with salt and pepper to taste and cook for 15 minutes, until the potatoes are tender. Mash the potatoes roughly in their liquid, then add the greens and boil uncovered for 10 minutes. Add the parsley and simmer for 2–3 minutes, until heated through. Serve with long croûtons.

Salads

Spinach, avocado and bacon salad

alcohol free ✓ | citrus free ✗ | dairy free ✓ | gluten free ✓ | wheat free ✓

Serves 4–6
Preparation time: 5 minutes
Cooking time: 8 minutes

Per serving
Energy 466 kcals/1920 kJ | Protein 10 g | Carbohydrate 6 g | Fat 45 g
Fibre 5 g

1 ripe avocado, peeled and pitted
2 tablespoons lemon juice
500 g (1 lb) young spinach leaves
1 small bunch spring onions, shredded into julienne strips
4 slices back bacon, rinded and chopped
1 garlic clove, crushed
1 quantity Walnut Dressing (see page 152)

1 Dice the avocado flesh and sprinkle with lemon juice to stop it discolouring. Make sure the spinach leaves are thoroughly rinsed and dry, then tear into pieces and put into a serving bowl, together with the spring onions and avocado cubes.

2 Dry-fry the bacon with the garlic in a heavy-based frying pan until crisp and brown and all the fat has been released. Remove with a slotted spoon, drain on kitchen paper, then scatter over the spinach mixture.

3 Spoon Walnut Dressing over the salad, toss gently to coat and serve at once.

Baby corn and alfalfa salad

alcohol free ✓ | citrus free ✗ | dairy free ✓ | gluten free ✓ | wheat free ✓

Serves 4–6
Preparation time: 15 minutes
Cooking time: 8–10 minutes

Per serving
Energy 200 kcals/840 kJ | Protein 7 g | Carbohydrate 4 g | Fat 18 g
Fibre 1 g

500 g (1 lb) baby corn cobs
125 g (4 oz) alfalfa sprouts
5 tablespoons light olive oil or groundnut oil
½ onion, chopped
25 g (1 oz) flaked almonds
2 tablespoons white wine vinegar
½ teaspoon finely grated lemon rind
½ teaspoon soft brown sugar
1 tablespoon chopped parsley
salt and pepper

1 Unless they are very small, halve the baby corn cobs lengthways. Add to a saucepan of boiling water and cook for about 3–4 minutes, until barely tender. Drain in a colander and refresh under cold running water. Drain again thoroughly and put into a large shallow bowl with the alfalfa sprouts.

2 Heat 2 tablespoons of the oil in a small frying pan, add the onion and cook for about 3 minutes, until softened. Transfer to a small bowl.

3 Add the almonds to the frying pan and cook, stirring, for 1–2 minutes, until lightly browned. Add to the onion with the remaining ingredients, including the oil. Stir well.

4 To serve, season the salad with salt and pepper. Spoon over the dressing mixture and toss lightly.

Celery, red onion and new potato salad

alcohol free ✓ | citrus free ✓ | dairy free ✓ | gluten free ✓ | wheat free ✓

Serves 4
Preparation time: 10 minutes
Cooking time: 10–15 minutes

Per serving
Energy 380 kcals/1577 kJ | Protein 4 g | Carbohydrate 26 g | Fat 30 g
Fibre 3 g

500 g (1 lb) new potatoes, halved
1 small fennel bulb, halved, cored and finely sliced
2 celery sticks, thinly sliced
1 red onion, halved and thinly sliced
celery leaves or dill sprigs, to garnish (optional)

Dressing:
150 ml (¼ pint) mayonnaise
2 teaspoons coarse-grain mustard
2 tablespoons finely chopped dill
salt and pepper

1 Add the potatoes to a large saucepan of boiling water and boil for 10–15 minutes or until they are tender.

2 Meanwhile, mix together the fennel, celery and onion in a large, shallow bowl and set aside.

3 To make the dressing, mix together the mayonnaise, mustard and dill in a small bowl and season to taste.

4 Drain the potatoes, rinse them under cold running water, then drain again. Add the potatoes to the salad. Add the dressing and toss the ingredients until they are well coated. Garnish with celery leaves or dill sprigs, if liked.

Grilled aubergine and courgette salad with honey-mint dressing

alcohol free ✓ I citrus free ✗ I dairy free ✗ I gluten free ✗ I wheat free ✗

Serves 4
Preparation time: 15 minutes
Cooking time: 4–6 minutes

Per serving
Energy 215 kcals/894 kJ I Protein 8 g I Carbohydrate 12 g I Fat 16 g
Fibre 3 g

2 medium aubergines, thinly sliced
2 courgettes, thinly sliced
1 red pepper, cored, deseeded and cut into strips
about 3 tablespoons olive oil
125 g (4 oz) feta cheese
mint leaves, to garnish
toasted flat breads or crusty baguette, to serve

Honey-mint dressing:
50 g (2 oz) mint leaves, coarsely chopped
1 tablespoon clear honey
1 teaspoon prepared English mustard
2 tablespoons lime juice
salt and pepper

1 Brush the aubergine and courgette slices, and red pepper strips with olive oil. Heat the grill on the hottest setting and grill the vegetables for 2–3 minutes on each side, until lightly cooked.

2 Arrange the grilled vegetables in a shallow dish. Crumble the feta cheese and sprinkle it over the vegetables.

3 Thoroughly mix the dressing ingredients in a small bowl, adding salt and pepper to taste. Pour the dressing over the salad.

4 Scatter the mint leaves over the salad as a garnish. Serve with toasted flat breads or crusty baguette.

Chinese noodle and prawn salad

alcohol free ✓ | citrus free ✓ | dairy free ✓ | gluten free ✗ | wheat free ✗

Serves 4–6
Preparation time: 15 minutes
Cooking time: about 6 minutes

Per serving
Energy 380 kcals/1590 kJ | Protein 18 g | Carbohydrate 38 g | Fat 18 g
Fibre 3 g

175 g (6 oz) Chinese dried egg noodles
6 spring onions
1 small bunch of radishes, trimmed
175 g (6 oz) sugar snap peas, topped and tailed
175 g (6 oz) cooked peeled prawns
1 quantity Ginger and Lime Dressing (see page 154) or Sweet and
  Sour Dressing (see page 153)
salt and pepper

1 Bring a saucepan of water to the boil, add the noodles, cover the pan and remove from the heat. Leave to stand for 5 minutes, until the noodles are just tender. Drain in a colander and cool under cold running water. Drain well and transfer to a salad bowl.

2 Meanwhile, cut the spring onions into short lengths and shred finely. Leave the radishes whole or cut them into slices, as preferred. Add both the shredded spring onions and the radishes to the noodles.

3 Bring a saucepan of water to the boil, add the sugar snap peas and blanch for 1 minute. Drain in a colander, refresh under cold running water and drain again. Add to the salad with the prawns. Season with salt and pepper.

4 Just before serving, add the chosen dressing to the salad and toss lightly.

Salade niçoise

alcohol free ✓ | citrus free ✗ | dairy free ✓ | gluten free ✓ | wheat free ✓

Serves 2 as a main course
Preparation time: 10 minutes
Cooking time: 15–18 minutes

Per serving
Energy 560 kcals/2340 kJ | Protein 36 g | Carbohydrate 27 g | Fat 35 g
Fibre 6 g

250 g (8 oz) small new potatoes, scrubbed, or medium potatoes,
   scrubbed and quartered
5 tablespoons virgin olive oil
2 tablespoons red wine vinegar
250 g (8 oz) French beans
250 g (8 oz) fresh tuna steak, cut into finger strips
2 garlic cloves, finely chopped
2 anchovy fillets, chopped
about 1½ teaspoons Dijon mustard
1 red pepper, charred, skinned,
   deseeded and thinly sliced
2 tablespoons capers
salt and pepper
lemon wedges, to serve (optional)

1 Steam the potatoes for 8–10 minutes, until just tender. Transfer to a serving bowl and toss gently with 1 tablespoon each of the oil and the vinegar. Season to taste with salt and pepper.

2 Steam the French beans for 5–6 minutes, until just tender. Set aside.

3 Heat 1 tablespoon of the oil in a nonstick frying pan. Add the tuna and sear evenly over a high heat. Add to the potato mixture.

4 Add the remaining oil to the frying pan, then stir in the garlic and anchovies for 30 seconds. Stir in the remaining vinegar and boil for about 1 minute. Stir in mustard to taste, then pour over the potato mixture. Add the pepper strips, beans, capers and more pepper. Toss gently, taste and adjust the flavourings if necessary, then serve the salad immediately with lemon wedges, if liked.

Walnut dressing

alcohol free ✓ I citrus free ✓ I dairy free ✓ I gluten free ✓ I wheat free ✓

Makes about 150 ml (¼ pint)
Preparation time: 10 minutes

Whole recipe
Energy 924 kcals/3800 kJ I Protein 3 g I Carbohydrate 6 g I Fat 99 g
Fibre 1 g

3 tablespoons balsamic vinegar
1 teaspoon soft light brown sugar
1 teaspoon Dijon mustard
125 ml (4 fl oz) walnut oil
1 tablespoon finely chopped walnuts
1 tablespoon chopped parsley or basil
salt and pepper

1 Combine the vinegar, sugar and mustard in a small bowl. Add salt and pepper to taste. Stir to mix, then gradually whisk in the walnut oil, using a balloon whisk.

2 Stir the chopped walnuts and herbs into the dressing and adjust the seasoning to taste.

Sweet and sour dressing

alcohol free ✓ | citrus free ✓ | dairy free ✓ | gluten free ✗ | wheat free ✗

Makes about 250 ml (8 fl oz)
Preparation time: 10 minutes

Whole recipe
Energy 565 kcals/2334 kJ | Protein 3 g | Carbohydrate 15 g | Fat 55 g
Fibre 2 g

1 spring onion
2 fresh ripe plums, pitted and finely diced
5 tablespoons olive or groundnut oil
2 tablespoons sherry vinegar
2 teaspoons soy sauce
2 teaspoons tomato purée
½ garlic clove, crushed
¼ teaspoon soft light brown sugar
salt and pepper

1 Cut the spring onion into fine shreds about 2.5 cm (1 inch) long. Put into a small bowl or screw-top jar. Add the diced plums.

2 Add the remaining ingredients to the bowl or jar and either whisk together with a fork or shake in the closed jar until combined. Use the dressing as required.

Ginger and lime dressing

alcohol free ✓ | citrus free ✗ | dairy free ✓ | gluten free ✓ | wheat free ✓

Makes about 150 ml (¼ pint)
Preparation time: 10 minutes

Whole recipe
Energy 583 kcals/2406 kJ | Protein 1 g | Carbohydrate 22 g | Fat 55 g
Fibre 0 g

2 teaspoons grated fresh root ginger
1 garlic clove, crushed
2 limes
1 tablespoon clear honey
75 ml (3 fl oz) groundnut or grapeseed oil
2 tablespoons chopped coriander
salt and pepper

1 Combine the ginger and garlic in a bowl. Grate the rind of the
limes finely and add to the bowl with the honey. Stir in salt and
pepper to taste.

2 Squeeze the juice from both limes. Add to the bowl and beat well
with a balloon whisk or wooden spoon. Pour in the oil, whisking
the dressing until well mixed. Alternatively, put the ingredients
into a screw-top jar and shake until thoroughly combined. Just
before using the dressing, stir in the chopped coriander.

Light lunches

Vegetable carpaccio with parmesan shavings

alcohol free ✓ | citrus free ✓ | dairy free ✗ | gluten free ✓ | wheat free ✓

Serves 4
Preparation time: 15 minutes

Per serving
Energy 85 kcals/350 kJ | Protein 4 g | Carbohydrate 6 g | Fat 5 g
Fibre 3 g

12 small radishes, trimmed and sliced
1 green pepper, cored, deseeded and cut into thin strips
1 red pepper, cored, deseeded and cut into thin strips
2 small carrots, thinly sliced
3 celery stalks, thinly sliced
1 small fennel bulb, thinly sliced
1 tablespoon extra virgin olive oil
25 g (1 oz) Parmesan cheese, shaved
pepper

1 Divide the vegetables between 4 large plates, and arrange them in attractive mounds in the centre.

2 Drizzle the vegetables with enough olive oil to lightly moisten them. Scatter the Parmesan shavings around them and garnish with a few grindings of black pepper.

Greek pitta wraps

alcohol free ✓ | citrus free ✓ | dairy free ✗ | gluten free ✗ | wheat free ✗

Makes 4
Preparation time: 10 minutes
Cooking time: 2–3 minutes

Per serving
Energy 560 kcals/2346 kJ | Protein 19 g | Carbohydrate 59 g | Fat 29 g
Fibre 5 g

4 large pitta breads
125 g (4 oz) cooked lamb, finely shredded
1 small bunch spring onions, trimmed and chopped
2 lettuce leaves, chopped
2 tomatoes, skinned, deseeded and chopped
4 black olives, halved and pitted
75 g (3 oz) feta cheese, crumbled
4 lettuce leaves
salt and pepper

Dressing:
2 tablespoons natural yogurt
2 tablespoons olive oil
¼ teaspoon Dijon mustard
¼ teaspoon clear honey
salt and pepper

1 Carefully cut a slit across the top of each pitta bread. Gently open out each bread so that they form a pocket. Mix the dressing ingredients together in a small bowl, and season with salt and pepper to taste.

2 Mix the lamb with the spring onions, chopped lettuce, tomatoes, olives, dressing and salt and pepper to taste, blending well.

3 Divide both the salad mixture and the feta equally among the pitta pockets.

4 Cook under a preheated moderate grill for about 2–3 minutes, until the filling is bubbling, turning once. Add the fresh lettuce leaves and quickly roll up the pittas in greaseproof paper.

Summer vegetables with herb aïoli

alcohol free ✓ | citrus free ✗ | dairy free ✓ | gluten free ✓ | wheat free ✓

Serves 4
Preparation time: 15 minutes

Per serving
Energy 565 kcals/2330 kJ | Protein 4 g | Carbohydrate 7 g | Fat 58 g
Fibre 2 g

500 g (1 lb) fresh summer vegetables
lemon wedges, to serve

Herb aïoli:
2–8 garlic cloves, depending on personal taste
½ teaspoon sea salt
2 egg yolks
1 tablespoon lemon juice
1 teaspoon Dijon mustard
300 ml (½ pint) French extra virgin olive oil
4 tablespoons mixed herbs, to include basil, chives and parsley
1–2 tablespoons boiling water (optional)
pepper

1 To make the aïoli, crush the garlic cloves with the sea salt in a
mortar or by pounding them together on a board with the side of
a knife blade. Put into a food processor with the egg yolks, lemon
juice, mustard and pepper and process briefly until pale.

2 Gradually pour in the oil through the feeder funnel until the sauce
is emulsified, thick and glossy. Add the herbs at the end. You may
need to thin the aïoli slightly by whisking in a little boiling water.

3 Wash the vegetables and pat dry. Arrange the vegetables on a
large platter and serve with lemon wedges and the herb aïoli.

Spanish tortilla

alcohol free ✓ | citrus free ✓ | dairy free ✓ | gluten free ✓ | wheat free ✓

Serves 10–12
Preparation time: 10 minutes
Cooking time: 45 minutes

Per serving
Energy 226 kcals/939 kJ | Protein 5 g | Carbohydrate 15 g | Fat 17 g
Fibre 2 g

200 ml (7 fl oz) extra virgin olive oil
750 g (1½ lb) waxy potatoes, cubed
1 onion, chopped
4 large eggs
salt and pepper

1 Heat the oil in a large frying pan, add the potatoes, onion and a little salt and fry over a low heat for about 20 minutes, stirring occasionally to prevent sticking.

2 Beat the eggs in a large bowl. Lift the potatoes and onions out of the pan with a slotted spoon and stir them into the beaten eggs, adding a little more salt and some pepper. Set aside to soak for 10 minutes. Pour off the oil, reserving 3 tablespoons.

3 Return 2 tablespoons of the oil to the pan and heat until hot. Add the potato mixture, reduce the heat and cook gently for about 10 minutes, until it is golden underneath and almost set. Carefully flip the tortilla on to a large plate so that the cooked side is on top. Add the remaining oil to the pan, ease the tortilla back in, and cook the second side for about 5 minutes.

4 Remove the tortilla from the frying pan. Serve warm or leave to cool, cut into squares or wedges.

Braised provençal artichokes

alcohol free ✗ | citrus free ✗ | dairy free ✗ | gluten free ✓ | wheat free ✓

Serves 4
Preparation time: 15 minutes
Cooking time: about 1 hour

Per serving
Energy 280 kcals/1164 kJ | Protein 6 g | Carbohydrate 11 g | Fat 23 g
Fibre 1 g

2 lemons, halved
4 large globe artichokes
8 tablespoons extra virgin olive oil
2 garlic cloves
2 shallots, finely chopped
1 teaspoon chopped thyme
50 g (2 oz) piece of smoked pancetta, diced
1 large ripe beef tomato, skinned and diced
1 tablespoon chopped basil
2 tablespoons dry white wine
salt and pepper
a little shaved Parmesan cheese, to serve
basil leaves, to garnish

1 Fill a large bowl with cold water and squeeze in the juice from half of one of the lemons. Snap off most of the stem from the artichokes leaving about 2.5 cm (1 inch). Peel away as many of the large tough leaves from around the base as possible and cut off a good 2.5 cm (1 inch) from the top. Rub all over with the second lemon half and put into the bowl of acidulated water.

2 Plunge the artichokes into a large pan of lightly salted boiling water, cover and simmer for about 20 minutes, until they feel tender. Transfer them to kitchen paper, inverting them to extract excess water, and leave until cool enough to handle.

3 Meanwhile, heat 2 tablespoons of the oil in a frying pan and gently fry the garlic, shallots and thyme for 5 minutes. Add the pancetta, fry until golden, then add the tomato and basil. Remove from the heat.

4 Cut the artichokes in half, scooping out and discarding the hairy chokes from the middle, and arrange, cut side up, in a large ovenproof dish. Spoon the tomato mixture into the hollow middles and over the stems, drizzle over the remaining oil and squeeze over the juice from half of the remaining lemon. Season liberally with salt and pepper. Add the wine to the dish, cover and bake in a preheated oven at 180°C (350°F), Gas Mark 4, for 30 minutes, until really tender.

5 Serve hot or warm, garnished with basil leaves and drizzled with plenty more olive oil, a squeeze of lemon juice and with Parmesan shavings.

Aubergine, tomato and feta rolls

alcohol free ✓ | citrus free ✓ | dairy free ✗ | gluten free ✓ | wheat free ✓

Serves 4
Preparation time: 15 minutes
Cooking time: about 6 minutes

Per serving
Energy 366 kcals/1514 kJ | Protein 8 g | Carbohydrate 5 g | Fat 35 g
Fibre 3 g

2 medium aubergines
3 tablespoons olive oil
125 g (4 oz) feta cheese, coarsely diced
12 sun-dried tomatoes in oil, drained
15–20 basil leaves
salt and pepper

1 Trim the ends off the aubergines, then cut off a thin slice
lengthways from both sides of each; discard these slices, which
should be mainly skin. Cut each aubergine lengthways into 4
slices. Heat the grill on the hottest setting or heat a griddle pan
on the hob.

2 Brush both sides of the aubergine slices with oil and grill them
for about 3 minutes on each side. Alternatively, cook them in
the griddle pan, turning once, until browned and softened.

3 Lay the aubergine slices on a board and divide the cheese,
tomatoes and basil leaves between them. Season well with
salt and pepper. Roll up the slices from the short ends and
secure them with cocktail sticks. Arrange on serving plates
and serve at once or cover and set aside in a cool place, but
not the refrigerator.

Courgette and mint frittata

alcohol free ✓ | citrus free ✓ | dairy free ✗ | gluten free ✓ | wheat free ✓

Serves 4
Preparation time: 10 minutes
Cooking time: 15–18 minutes

Per serving
Energy 287 kcals/1193 kJ | Protein 16 g | Carbohydrate 11 g | Fat 21 g
Fibre 1 g

2 tablespoons olive oil
1 red onion, thinly sliced
500 g (1 lb) courgettes, thinly sliced
1 red chilli, deseeded and thinly sliced
5 eggs, beaten
1 tablespoon double cream
4 tablespoons chopped mint
50 g (2 oz) Parmesan cheese, grated
salt and pepper

1 Heat the oil in a 20 cm (8 inch) frying pan. Add the onion and cook over a moderate heat for about 3–4 minutes, stirring, until softened slightly. Add the courgettes and the chilli, then increase the heat to high and cook for 4–5 minutes.

2 Meanwhile, beat the eggs with the cream, adding salt and pepper and mint. Pour the eggs over the mixture. Reduce the heat to medium and cook for about 5 minutes, until the eggs are just set on top and golden underneath. Use a spatula or fish slice to lift the edge to check that it is browned underneath.

3 Sprinkle the Parmesan over the frittata and put it under a hot grill for 3–4 minutes, until the frittata is golden and set. Cut into wedges and serve.

Grilled chicory with salsa verde

alcohol free ✓ I citrus free ✕ I dairy free ✕ I gluten free ✕ I wheat free ✕

Serves 4
Preparation time: 15 minutes
Cooking time: 9 minutes

Per serving
Energy 570 kcals/2359 kJ I Protein 17 g I Carbohydrate 6 g I Fat 55 g
Fibre 5 g

4 heads of treviso or chicory, each about 150 g (5 oz), trimmed and
    halved lengthways
2 tablespoons olive oil
125 g (4 oz) Parmesan cheese, coarsely grated
chopped parsley, to garnish
toasted ciabatta bread, to serve

Salsa verde:
200 g (7 oz) flat leaf parsley
50 g (2 oz) pine nuts, toasted
2 pickled gherkins
8 green olives, pitted
1 garlic clove, chopped
1 tablespoon lemon juice
150 ml (¼ pint) olive oil
salt and pepper

1 First make the salsa verde: coarsely purée all the ingredients, except the oil, in a food processor or blender. With the motor still running, gradually trickle in the oil to make a creamy paste. Transfer to a serving dish, cover and set aside. (The salsa will keep for up to 1 week in the refrigerator.)

2 Heat the grill on the hottest setting. Put the treviso or chicory halves onto the grill rack, cut sides down, brush with some of the oil and grill for 5 minutes. Turn the vegetables, brush with the remaining oil and sprinkle the Parmesan over the top. Grill for a further 4 minutes, until the cheese has melted and the edges begin to char.

3 Transfer the treviso or chicory to plates and garnish with chopped parsley. Add a little salsa verde to each plate and serve immediately, offering the remaining salsa verde separately. Toasted ciabatta bread is a good accompaniment.

Main dishes

Seared scallops with carrot, papaya and red onion salad

alcohol free ✓ I citrus free ✕ I dairy free ✓ I gluten free ✓ I wheat free ✓

Serves 4
Preparation time: 15 minutes
Cooking time: 2–4 minutes

Per serving
Energy 230 kcals/967 kJ I Protein 28 g I Carbohydrate 12 g I Fat 8 g
Fibre 3 g

1 small green papaya or 1 cucumber
1 carrot, finely shredded
1 red onion, thinly sliced
50 g (2 oz) roasted peanuts
2 tablespoons lime juice
1 tablespoon Thai fish sauce (nam pla)
4 tablespoons finely chopped coriander leaves
12 large or king scallops, cleaned
salt and pepper
chilli oil, to serve (optional)

1 Halve the papaya, scoop out the seeds, then peel the flesh. If using a cucumber, halve it lengthways and scoop out the seeds, then peel it thinly. Finely shred the prepared papaya or cucumber.

2 Mix the papaya or cucumber with the carrot, onion and peanuts. Stir in the lime juice, fish sauce and coriander. Divide this salad among 4 serving plates.

3 Slice the scallops in half horizontally. Heat a large, nonstick frying pan until very hot. Add the scallops and cook them for 1–2 minutes on each side. Remove the pan from the heat and season the scallops with salt and pepper. Arrange the scallops around the salads and serve immediately, offering chilli oil separately for those who may want to spice up the salad.

Seared tuna with muhammara

alcohol free ✓ I citrus free ✗ I dairy free ✓ I gluten free ✗ I wheat free ✗

Serves 4
Preparation time: 35 minutes, including marinating
Cooking time: 10 minutes

Per serving
Energy 350 kcals/1460 kJ I Protein 20 g I Carbohydrate 4 g I Fat 28 g
Fibre 1 g

4 tuna steaks, about 175 g (6 oz) each
1 bunch of thyme
extra virgin olive oil
salt and pepper
rocket salad, to serve

Muhammara:
50 g (2 oz) walnuts
25 g (1 oz) fresh breadcrumbs
2 garlic cloves, crushed
1 tablespoon lemon juice
2 teaspoons pomegranate syrup
75 ml (3 fl oz) extra virgin olive oil
1–2 tablespoons boiling water
salt and pepper

1 Wash and dry the tuna and, using the thyme sprigs, rub all over with oil. Season well with salt and pepper and set aside.

2 To make the muhammara, put the walnuts, breadcrumbs, garlic, lemon juice, pomegranate syrup and salt and pepper into a food processor and pulse to form a fairly rough paste. Gradually blend in the oil until the sauce is amalgamated and fairly fine, adding a little boiling water to thin it slightly (it should have the texture of hummus). Taste and adjust the seasoning. Transfer the sauce to a bowl, cover with clingfilm and leave to infuse for 30 minutes.

3 Heat a ridged griddle pan until really hot (this will take about 3 minutes), then add the tuna steaks and cook for 1–2 minutes on each side. Transfer the steaks to a plate, cover with foil and leave to rest for 3–4 minutes. Serve with the muhammara and a rocket salad.

Sesame prawns with pak choi

alcohol free ✓ | citrus free ✗ | dairy free ✓ | gluten free ✗ | wheat free ✗

Serves 4
Preparation time: 5 minutes, plus marinating
Cooking time: 4–5 minutes

Per serving
Energy 165 kcals/690 kJ | Protein 16 g | Carbohydrate 9 g | Fat 8 g
Fibre 0 g

600 g (1 lb 3 oz) raw tiger prawns, peeled, with the tails left on
1 teaspoon sesame oil
2 tablespoons light soy sauce
1 tablespoon clear honey
1 teaspoon grated fresh root ginger
1 teaspoon crushed garlic
1 tablespoon lemon juice
500 g (1 lb) pak choi, heads cut in half lengthways
2 tablespoons vegetable oil
salt and pepper

1 Put the prawns, sesame oil, soy sauce, honey, ginger, garlic and lemon juice into a bowl. Season, mix well, then set aside.

2 Bring a large saucepan of water to a rolling boil. Blanch the pak choi halves in the boiling water for 40–50 seconds. Drain well, cover and keep warm.

3 Heat the oil in a large wok or frying pan. Add the prawns with their marinade and stir-fry briskly for 3–4 minutes, until the prawns are pink and just cooked through.

4 Divide the pak choi among 4 plates, then top with the prawns and any juices from the pan. Serve at once.

Mediterranean fish stew

alcohol free ✕ | citrus free ✓ | dairy free ✓ | gluten free ✓ | wheat free ✓

Serves 6
Preparation time: 15 minutes
Cooking time: 40 minutes

Per serving
Energy 259 kcals/1087 kJ | Protein 33 g | Carbohydrate 6 g | Fat 11 g
Fibre 1 g

3 tablespoons extra virgin olive oil
2 onions, sliced
2 carrots, sliced
3 celery sticks, sliced
125 g (4 oz) mushrooms
2 garlic cloves, crushed
4 tomatoes, skinned and chopped
300 ml (½ pint) dry white wine
600 ml (1 pint) fish or vegetable stock
750 g (1½ lb) cod or haddock fillet, skinned and boned
200 g (7 oz) jar mussels in brine, drained
175 g (6 oz) peeled prawns
salt and pepper

1 Heat the oil in a large saucepan and add the onions, carrots, celery, mushrooms and garlic. Cooked until softened, but not brown. Add the tomatoes, wine and stock. Season with salt and pepper to taste and simmer for 15 minutes.

2 Cut the fish into 5 cm (2 inch) cubes. Add them to the saucepan and simmer for 15 minutes.

3 Add the mussels and prawns and simmer for 2–3 minutes. Serve in a warmed serving dish.

Pea and prawn risotto

alcohol free ✗ | citrus free ✓ | dairy free ✗ | gluten free ✓ | wheat free ✓

Serves 6
Preparation time: 10 minutes
Cooking time: 30 minutes

Per serving
Energy 407 kcals/1700 kJ | Protein 14 g | Carbohydrate 44 g | Fat 19 g
Fibre 6 g

500 g (1 lb) raw prawns
125 g (4 oz) butter
1 onion, finely chopped
2 garlic cloves, crushed
250 g (8 oz) risotto rice
375 g (12 oz) shelled peas
150 ml (¼ pint) dry white wine
1.5 litres (2½ pints) vegetable stock
4 tablespoons chopped mint
salt and pepper

1 Peel and devein the prawns, reserving the heads and shells. Wash the heads and shells and pat dry.

2 Melt half of the butter in a large frying pan, add the heads and shells and stir-fry for 3–4 minutes, until golden. Strain the butter and return it to the pan.

3 Add a further 25 g (1 oz) of the butter to the pan and fry the onion and garlic for 5 minutes until softened. Add the rice and stir for 1 minute, until coated. Add the peas and wine and boil rapidly until reduced by half.

4 Meanwhile, bring the stock to a very gentle simmer in another pan. Gradually add it to the rice, a ladleful at a time, stirring constantly until the rice is creamy but still crunchy in the middle and most of the liquid has been absorbed. This takes about 20 minutes.

5 Stir-fry the prawns in the remaining butter for 3–4 minutes, then stir into the rice with the mint and salt and pepper. Cover and leave for 5 minutes. Serve hot.

Prawn and monkfish ravioli

alcohol free ✓ I citrus free ✗ I dairy free ✗ I gluten free ✗ I wheat free ✗

Serves 4
Preparation time: 30 minutes, plus chilling
Cooking time: 12 minutes

Per serving
Energy 425 kcals/1790 kJ I Protein 28 g I Carbohydrate 57 g I Fat 14 g
Fibre 3 g

250 g (8 oz) raw prawns, peeled, deveined and finely chopped
250 g (8 oz) monkfish fillet, finely chopped
2 tablespoons chopped parsley, plus extra for garnishing
1 teaspoon grated lime rind
4 tablespoons single cream
salt and pepper
flat leaf parsley sprigs, to garnish

Pepper butter:
½ large red pepper, cored and deseeded
25 g (1 oz) low-fat spread
1 tablespoon lime juice

Pasta:
250 g (8 oz) pasta flour (or plain flour), plus extra for dusting
1 teaspoon salt
2 eggs, plus 1 egg yolk
1 tablespoon olive oil

1 To make the pepper butter, grill the pepper for 3–4 minutes on each side until charred and tender. Seal in a plastic bag until cool. Discard the skin and purée the flesh in a food processor or blender with the low-fat spread and lime juice until smooth. Season with salt and pepper to taste.

2 Make the pasta dough. Sift the flour and salt into a bowl, and work in the eggs, egg yolk, oil and enough water to form a soft dough. Knead the dough for 5 minutes until smooth; wrap and chill for 30 minutes.

3 Meanwhile, make the filling. Mix the prawns and monkfish with the parsley, lime rind and cream. Season with salt and pepper and set aside.

4 Divide the dough into 8 portions. Roll out each piece thinly on a floured surface. Take one sheet of pasta and place teaspoons of the filling at 2.5 cm (1 inch) intervals on the dough. Brush lightly around the filling with water and top with a second sheet of pasta. Press down around each mound and, using a pastry cutter, stamp out the ravioli. Repeat with the remaining mixture, placing the filled ravioli on a well-floured dish towel.

5 Add the ravioli to a large saucepan of lightly salted boiling water and boil for 3–4 minutes, then drain well. Serve with pepper butter and garnish with chopped parsley and sprigs of flat leaf parsley.

Baked sea bass with fennel and green olives

alcohol free ✗ | citrus free ✗ | dairy free ✓ | gluten free ✓ | wheat free ✓

Serves 4
Preparation time: 15 minutes
Cooking time: 35 minutes

Per serving
Energy 556 kcals/2316 kJ | Protein 52 g | Carbohydrate 2 g | Fat 36 g
Fibre 1 g

1.25 kg (2½ lb) sea bass, scaled and gutted
a few rosemary sprigs
2 large fennel bulbs
150 ml (¼ pint) good olive oil
4 tablespoons lemon juice
1 tablespoon dried oregano
3 tablespoons chopped parsley
8 large green olives, pitted
150 ml (¼ pint) dry white wine
salt and pepper
fennel fronds, to garnish

1 Wash the fish inside and out and pat dry with kitchen paper. Fill the cavity with sprigs of rosemary.

2 Cut the fennel bulbs in half lengthways, cut out the core and slice thickly. Blanch in boiling salted water for 5 minutes. Drain.

3 Whisk together the oil, lemon juice, oregano, parsley and salt and pepper in a bowl and stir in the fennel, to coat. Tip this mixture into a shallow, oval ovenproof dish that will take the fish as well. Lay the fish on top of the fennel and pour over any remaining liquid. Tuck in the olives and pour over the wine.

4 Bake the fish in a preheated oven at 220°C (425°F), Gas Mark 7, for 30 minutes. Open the oven and spoon the juices over the fish and stir the fennel around. Turn off the oven, leaving the fish to set for 5 minutes, and then serve immediately, garnished with fennel fronds.

Grilled swordfish with toasted almond and parsley pesto

alcohol free ✓ | citrus free ✕ | dairy free ✕ | gluten free ✓ | wheat free ✓

Serves 4
Preparation time: 10 minutes
Cooking time: 10 minutes

Per serving
Energy 754 kcals/3124 kJ | Protein 43 g | Carbohydrate 3 g | Fat 64 g
Fibre 5 g

125 g (4 oz) unblanched whole almonds
1 garlic clove, crushed
2 tablespoons freshly grated Parmesan cheese
50 g (2 oz) parsley, roughly chopped
200 ml (7 fl oz) extra virgin olive oil
2 tablespoons fresh ricotta cheese
4 swordfish steaks about 175 g (6 oz) each
olive oil, for brushing
salt and pepper
lemon wedges, to garnish

1 Spread the almonds on a baking sheet and put it under a preheated grill for 2–3 minutes, turning the almonds often until they are toasted and golden. (You may have to break one open to see.)

2 Put half of the toasted almonds into a food processor or blender with the garlic, Parmesan, parsley, olive oil, ricotta and salt and pepper and blend until smooth, scraping down the sides of the bowl if necessary. Roughly chop the remaining almonds and stir them into the pesto.

3 Brush the swordfish steaks with olive oil and cook under a preheated hot grill for 2–3 minutes on each side, until just cooked through. Season with salt and pepper and serve the fish with the pesto, garnished with lemon wedges.

Salmon steaks in fresh coriander sauce

alcohol free ✕ | citrus free ✕ | dairy free ✕ | gluten free ✓ | wheat free ✓

Serves 4
Preparation time: 10 minutes
Cooking time: 40 minutes

Per serving
Energy 758 kcals/3136 kJ | Protein 38 g | Carbohydrate 4 g | Fat 66 g
Fibre 1 g

4 salmon steaks, 175–250 g (6–8 oz) each
125 g (4 oz) unsalted butter, plus extra for greasing
½ onion, finely chopped
1 carrot, cut into matchstick strips
1 garlic clove, finely chopped
1 bay leaf
1 tablespoon dry vermouth (optional)
125 ml (4 fl oz) fish stock
1 bunch of coriander, finely chopped
125 ml (4 fl oz) double cream
1–2 tablespoons lemon juice
sea salt and pepper
lime wedges, to garnish
freshly cooked vegetables, such as new potatoes and
    French beans, to serve

1 Rinse the salmon steaks in cold water, pat dry and season with salt and pepper.

2 Melt half the butter in a small frying pan. Add the onion and carrot and sauté over a low heat for 4–5 minutes. Add the garlic and cook for a further 2 minutes.

3 Pour into a shallow ovenproof dish, add the bay leaf, then arrange the fish on top in a single layer. Sprinkle with vermouth, if using, then with the fish stock. Cover with buttered foil and bake in a preheated oven at 190°C (375°F), Gas Mark 5, for 20–25 minutes, depending on the thickness of the fish. It should just flake easily when tested with a fork.

4 Remove the fish to a warmed serving plate and keep warm.

5 Strain the cooking juices into a clean pan and boil vigorously for 1–2 minutes to reduce.

6 Add half the remaining butter, the coriander and the cream, and simmer for 4–5 minutes, until slightly thickened. Add the lemon juice, stir for 1 minute, then add the remaining butter and whisk until smooth and glossy. Adjust the seasoning, if necessary, then pour the sauce over the fish. Garnish with the lime wedges and serve with vegetables.

Grilled cod steaks with mint pesto

alcohol free ✓ | citrus free ✕ | dairy free ✕ | gluten free ✓ | wheat free ✓

Serves 4
Preparation time: 10 minutes
Cooking time: about 8 minutes

Per serving
Energy 223 kcals/929 kJ | Protein 29 g | Carbohydrate 1 g | Fat 12 g
Fibre 0 g

4 cod steaks, about 175 g (6 oz) each
olive oil, for brushing
lemon juice
salt and pepper
lime wedges, to garnish

Mint pesto:
6 tablespoons chopped mint
1 tablespoon chopped parsley
1 garlic clove, chopped
1 tablespoon grated Parmesan cheese
1 tablespoon single cream
1 teaspoon balsamic vinegar
3 tablespoons extra virgin olive oil

1 Brush the cod with oil and squeeze over a little lemon juice. Season with salt and pepper and cook under a preheated moderate grill for 3–4 minutes on each side, until golden and cooked through.

2 Meanwhile, put all the ingredients for the pesto into a food processor or blender and blend until fairly smooth. Season with salt and pepper to taste and transfer to a bowl. Alternatively, pound the ingredients together with a mortar and pestle.

3 Serve the cod steaks topped with a spoonful of the pesto and green beans, if liked. Garnish with lime wedges.

Red mullet with mint sauce

alcohol free ✓ | citrus free ✗ | dairy free ✓ | gluten free ✗ | wheat free ✗

Serves 6
Preparation time: 10 minutes
Cooking time: 2–6 minutes

Per serving
Energy 320 kcals/1329 kJ | Protein 19 g | Carbohydrate 6 g | Fat 25 g
Fibre 1 g

50 g (2 oz) stale breadcrumbs
3 tablespoons white wine vinegar
3 tablespoons chopped mint
3 tablespoons chopped parsley
1 tablespoon salted capers, rinsed
1 egg, beaten
2 teaspoons sugar
2 teaspoons anchovy paste or 2 anchovy fillets, drained and
    roughly chopped
150 ml (¼ pint) fruity olive oil, plus extra for frying
1 kg (2 lb) small red mullet, cleaned and scaled
seasoned flour, for coating
salt and pepper

To garnish:
lemon wedges
mint sprigs

1 Moisten the breadcrumbs with 2 tablespoons of the vinegar and a little water. Let the breadcrumbs stand for a couple of minutes, then squeeze out the moisture.

2 Put the breadcrumbs into a food processor and add the mint, parsley, capers, egg, sugar and anchovy paste or fillets. Blend until smooth. With the machine running, gradually add the oil in a steady stream as if you were making mayonnaise. Taste and season with salt and pepper, then add the remaining vinegar if necessary. The sauce should be pale green and slightly sweet and sour. Transfer to a bowl.

3 Lightly coat the fish in seasoned flour and fry for 1–3 minutes on each side, until golden. Arrange the fish on a warmed platter and garnish with lemon wedges and mint sprigs. Serve the sauce separately.

Mussels alla marinara

alcohol free ✕ | citrus free ✓ | dairy free ✓ | gluten free ✕ | wheat free ✕

Serves 4
Preparation time: 15 minutes
Cooking time: 10 minutes

Per serving
Energy 249 kcals/1049 kJ | Protein 27 g | Carbohydrate 4 g | Fat 11 g
Fibre 1 g

2 kg (4 lb) fresh mussels
3 tablespoons olive oil
4 garlic cloves, chopped
150 ml (¼ pint) dry white wine
400 g (13 oz) can chopped tomatoes
1 small fresh red chilli, deseeded and finely chopped
4 tablespoons chopped parsley
salt and pepper
crusty bread, to serve

1 Scrub the mussels and remove the beards. Wash them in several changes of water and discard any that are not firmly closed.

2 Heat the oil in a large saucepan and fry the garlic until golden. Add the wine, tomatoes, chilli and half of the parsley and bring to the boil. Season well with salt and pepper, add the mussels and cover the pan. Cook over a brisk heat, shaking the pan, until all the mussels are open. Stir well. Discard any mussels that have not opened.

3 To serve, scatter the remaining parsley over the mussels and serve with crusty bread.

Lamb and courgette koftas

alcohol free ✓ | citrus free ✓ | dairy free ✓ | gluten free ✓ | wheat free ✓

Serves 4
Preparation time: 20 minutes
Cooking time: 5 minutes each batch

Per serving
Energy 203 kcals/849 kJ | Protein 16 g | Carbohydrate 5 g | Fat 14 g
Fibre 0 g

2 courgettes, finely grated
2 tablespoons sesame seeds
250 g (8 oz) minced lamb
2 spring onions, finely chopped
1 garlic clove, crushed
1 tablespoon chopped mint
½ teaspoon ground mixed spice
2 tablespoons dried breadcrumbs
1 egg, lightly beaten
vegetable oil, for shallow-frying
salt and pepper

1 Put the courgettes into a sieve and press to extract as much liquid as possible. Put into a bowl.

2 Dry-fry the sesame seeds in a heavy-based frying pan for 1–2 minutes, until they are golden and release their aroma. Add to the courgettes, together with the lamb and all the remaining ingredients, except the oil and lemon wedges. Season liberally with salt and pepper.

3 Form the mixture into 20 small balls and shallow-fry in batches for 5 minutes, turning frequently, until evenly browned. Keep the koftas warm while you are cooking the rest. Serve hot.

Lamb with piquant sauce

alcohol free ✓ | citrus free ✓ | dairy free ✓ | gluten free ✕ | wheat free ✕

Serves 4
Preparation time: 15 minutes, plus marinating
Cooking time: 10–15 minutes

Per serving
Energy 244 kcals/1020 kJ | Protein 29 g | Carbohydrate 5 g | Fat 13 g
Fibre 0 g

8 lamb cutlets, trimmed
8 tablespoons Worcestershire sauce
2 beef stock cubes
2 teaspoons chopped rosemary
1 teaspoon ground coriander
125 ml (4 fl oz) water
salt and pepper
rosemary sprigs, to garnish

To serve:
boiled rice (optional)
mangetout (optional)

1 Put the lamb cutlets into a flameproof dish. Put the Worcestershire sauce into a small bowl, crumble in the stock cubes and stir in the rosemary and coriander. Pour the mixture over the lamb, cover and leave to marinate for at least 3 hours, turning frequently.

2 Remove the lamb from the marinade and cook under a preheated hot grill for 10 minutes, until the lamb is cooked to your taste. Turn the meat frequently, spooning over some of the marinade to prevent the meat burning.

3 Put the remaining marinade into a saucepan along with the water and salt and pepper to taste. Bring to the boil. Arrange the lamb cutlets on warmed serving plates. Pour over the sauce and serve with boiled rice and mangetout, if liked, and garnish with rosemary sprigs.

Hot thai beef salad

alcohol free ✓ | citrus free ✗ | dairy free ✓ | gluten free ✓ | wheat free ✓

Serves 4
Preparation time: 15 minutes
Cooking time: 5 minutes

Per serving
Energy 290 kcals/1220 kJ | Protein 29 g | Carbohydrate 15 g | Fat 14 g
Fibre 4 g

2 ripe papayas, deseeded, peeled and thinly sliced
½ large cucumber, cut into matchsticks
75 g (3 oz) bean sprouts
2 spring onions, sliced lengthways
1 medium head crisp lettuce, shredded
2 tablespoons vegetable oil
500 g (1 lb) rump or fillet steak, cut into thin strips across the grain
3 garlic cloves, finely chopped
2 green chillies, thinly sliced
8 tablespoons lemon juice
1 tablespoon Thai fish sauce (nam pla)
2 teaspoons sugar

1 Arrange the papaya, cucumber, bean sprouts, spring onions and lettuce in separate piles on a large serving platter. Cover loosely and set aside.

2 Heat the oil in a heavy-based wok or frying pan over a moderate heat until hot. Add the beef, garlic and chillies, increase the heat to high and stir-fry for 3–4 minutes, until browned on all sides. Pour in the lemon juice and fish sauce, add the sugar and stir-fry until sizzling.

3 Arrange a bed of bean sprouts and lettuce on 4 serving plates. Remove the beef from the dressing with a slotted spoon and arrange on the salad. Arrange the papaya on one side and the cucumber and spring onion on top. Pour over the dressing and serve immediately.

Fusilli with broad beans, parma ham and mint

alcohol free ✕ | citrus free ✓ | dairy free ✕ | gluten free ✕ | wheat free ✕

Serves 4
Preparation time: 10 minutes
Cooking time: 15 minutes

Per serving
Energy 715 kcals/3000 kJ | Protein 30 g | Carbohydrate 87 g | Fat 27 g
Fibre 5 g

500 g (1 lb) shelled broad beans
375 g (12 oz) dried fusilli or other pasta shapes
4 tablespoons extra virgin olive oil
2 garlic cloves, finely chopped
150 ml (¼ pint) dry white wine
200 ml (7 fl oz) single cream
2 tablespoons chopped mint
4 slices of Parma ham, cut into thin strips
25 g (1 oz) pecorino sardo or Parmesan cheese,
    freshly grated, plus extra to serve
salt and pepper

1 Plunge the beans into a large saucepan of lightly salted boiling water and boil for 1 minute. Drain the beans and immediately refresh under cold water. Carefully peel away and discard the outer skins of the beans.

2 Cook the pasta in lightly salted boiling water, according to the packet instructions, until just tender.

3 Meanwhile, heat the oil in a deep frying pan and gently fry the garlic until softened but not browned. Add the wine, boil rapidly until it is reduced to about 2 tablespoons, then stir in the cream, mint and pepper to taste and heat through.

4 Drain the pasta and add to the sauce with the beans, Parma ham and pecorino or Parmesan. Stir over the heat for about 30 seconds and serve with extra cheese.

Penne with chicken livers

alcohol free ✓ | citrus free ✓ | dairy free ✕ | gluten free ✕ | wheat free ✕

Serves 4
Preparation time: 10 minutes
Cooking time: 10–15 minutes

Per serving
Energy 433 kcals/1826 kJ | Protein 23 g | Carbohydrate 60 g | Fat 13 g
Fibre 5 g

1 yellow pepper, cored and deseeded
300 g (10 oz) dried penne
1 tablespoon olive oil
25 g (1 oz) butter
1 red onion, sliced
250 g (8 oz) chicken livers, trimmed
1 rosemary sprig, chopped
salt and pepper
25 g (1 oz) grated Parmesan cheese, to serve

1 Roast the yellow pepper in a hot oven or under a preheated hot grill, skin-side up, until the skin is blistered and black. Put into a polythene bag and allow to cool, then peel off the skin. Cut the flesh into strips.

2 Cook the penne in lightly salted boiling water, according to the packet instructions, until just tender.

3 Meanwhile, heat the oil and butter in a large frying pan, add the onion and chicken livers and cook over high heat until browned all over – the livers are best eaten when still pink in the middle. Add the rosemary, the yellow pepper strips and salt and pepper to taste.

4 Mix the chicken liver mixture with the cooked pasta and toss well. Serve immediately with the Parmesan.

Fruit and nut couscous with chicken skewers

alcohol free ✓ | citrus free ✗ | dairy free ✓ | gluten free ✗ | wheat free ✗

Serves 4
Preparation time: 10 minutes, plus marinating
Cooking time: 20 minutes

Per serving
Energy 534 kcals/2228 kJ | Protein 34 g | Carbohydrate 39 g | Fat 28 g
Fibre 6 g

500 g (1 lb) free-range skinless chicken breast fillets, cut into long
   thin strips
2 tablespoons extra virgin olive oil
2 garlic cloves, crushed
½ teaspoon each ground cumin, turmeric and paprika
2 teaspoons lemon juice

Couscous:
4 tablespoons extra virgin olive oil
1 small onion, finely chopped
1 garlic clove, crushed
1 teaspoon each ground cumin, cinnamon, pepper and ginger
50 g (2 oz) dried dates, chopped
50 g (2 oz) dried apricots, finely chopped
50 g (2 oz) blanched almonds, toasted and chopped
600 ml (1 pint) vegetable stock
175 g (6 oz) couscous
1 tablespoon lemon juice
2 tablespoons chopped coriander
salt and pepper

1 Put the chicken strips into a shallow dish. Add the oil, garlic, spices and lemon juice. Stir well, then cover the dish and leave to marinate for 2 hours. Thread the chicken onto 8 small, presoaked wooden skewers.

2 To prepare the couscous, heat half of the oil in a saucepan and fry the onion, garlic and spices for 5 minutes. Stir in the dried fruits and almonds and remove from the heat.

3 Meanwhile, pour the stock over the couscous, cover with a tea towel and steam for 8–10 minutes, until the grains are fluffed up and the liquid absorbed. Stir in the remaining oil and the fruit and nut mixture. Add the lemon juice and coriander and season to taste with salt and pepper.

4 While the couscous is steaming, griddle or grill the chicken skewers for 4–5 minutes on each side, until charred and cooked through. Serve with the couscous.

Grilled chicken sala thai style

alcohol free ✓ I citrus free ✓ I dairy free ✓ I gluten free ✕ I wheat free ✕

Serves 4
Preparation time: 15 minutes, plus marinating
Cooking time: 20–30 minutes

Per serving
Energy 243 kcals/1020 kJ I Protein 27 g I Carbohydrate 16 g I Fat 8 g
Fibre 0 g

2 tablespoons crushed garlic
2 tablespoons chopped coriander root or stem
½ teaspoon pepper
1 teaspoon salt
2 tablespoons dark soy sauce
3 tablespoons honey
2 teaspoons ground ginger
1 tablespoon oyster sauce
8 chicken drumsticks, skinned and pierced with a fork
boiled rice, to serve (optional)

To garnish:
½ large red chilli, thinly sliced
2 spring onions, sliced into strips
2 teaspoons toasted sesame seeds

1 Put the crushed garlic, chopped coriander root or stem and the pepper into a food processor or blender and blend to a paste. Alternatively, pound together using a mortar and pestle.

2 Put the garlic mixture and the remaining ingredients into a flameproof dish large enough to hold the chicken drumsticks in a single layer. Coat the chicken well in the marinade, cover and set aside for 2 hours.

3 Grill the marinated drumsticks under a preheated, medium hot grill or on a barbecue for 20–30 minutes, turning frequently, until cooked through. Serve with boiled rice, if liked, and garnish with the chilli, spring onions and toasted sesame seeds.

Penne with broad beans, asparagus and mint

alcohol free ✓ I citrus free ✓ I dairy free ✗ I gluten free ✗ I wheat free ✗

Serves 4
Preparation time: 10 minutes
Cooking time: 20 minutes

Per serving
Energy 464 kcals/1950 kJ I Protein 22 g I Carbohydrate 64 g I Fat 15 g
Fibre 6 g

300 g (10 oz) dried penne
500 g (1 lb) asparagus, trimmed and cut into 5 cm (2 inch) lengths
2 tablespoons olive oil (optional)
250 g (8 oz) shelled broad beans or peas
75 ml (3 fl oz) half-fat crème fraîche
50 g (2 oz) Parmesan cheese, grated, plus extra to garnish
4 tablespoons chopped mint, plus extra to garnish
salt and pepper

1 Cook the pasta in lightly salted boiling water, according to the packet instructions, until just tender.

2 Meanwhile, steam the asparagus for 10–12 minutes. Alternatively, place it on a baking sheet, brush with olive oil and put under a preheated hot grill for 8 minutes, turning as the pieces brown.

3 Cook the broad beans or peas in lightly salted boiling water for 2 minutes, until tender.

4 Drain the pasta. Pour the crème fraîche into the empty pasta pan over the heat and add the beans or peas, asparagus and Parmesan. Heat gently and season with salt and pepper to taste. Return the pasta to the pan, add the mint and toss well with two wooden spoons. Serve immediately, garnished with Parmesan and mint.

Summer vegetable fettuccine

alcohol free ✓ | citrus free ✗ | dairy free ✗ | gluten free ✗ | wheat free ✗

Serves 4
Preparation time: 10 minutes
Cooking time: 17–23 minutes

Per serving

Energy 466 kcals/1975 kJ | Protein 23 g | Carbohydrate 81 g | Fat 8 g
Fibre 7 g

250 g (8 oz) asparagus, trimmed and cut into 5 cm (2 inch) lengths
125 g (4 oz) sugar snap peas, topped and tailed
400 g (13 oz) dried fettuccine or pappardelle
200 g (7 oz) baby courgettes
150 g (5 oz) button mushrooms
1 tablespoon olive oil
1 small onion, finely chopped
1 garlic clove, finely chopped
4 tablespoons lemon juice
2 teaspoons chopped tarragon
2 teaspoons chopped parsley
100 g (3½ oz) smoked mozzarella cheese, diced
salt and pepper
garlic bread, to serve

1 Bring a saucepan of water to the boil. Add the asparagus and sugar snap peas and boil for 3–4 minutes, then drain and refresh with cold water. Drain well and set aside.

2 Cook the fettuccine or pappardelle in a large saucepan of boiling salted water for 8–10 minutes or, according to the packet instructions, until just tender.

3 Meanwhile, halve the courgettes lengthways and cut the mushrooms in half. Heat the oil in a large frying pan. Add the onion and garlic and cook gently for about 2–3 minutes. Add the courgettes and mushrooms and fry, stirring, for 3–4 minutes. Stir in the asparagus and sugar snap peas and cook for 1–2 minutes then add the lemon juice, tarragon and parsley.

4 Drain the pasta and return it to the pan. Add the vegetable mixture and mozzarella and season to taste. Toss lightly to mix, then serve at once with garlic bread.

Beetroot risotto

alcohol free ✓ | citrus free ✓ | dairy free ✗ | gluten free ✓ | wheat free ✓

Serves 4
Preparation time: 5–10 minutes
Cooking time: about 23–24 minutes

Per serving
Energy 770 kcals/3241 kJ | Protein 12 g | Carbohydrate 118 g | Fat 31 g
Fibre 5 g

1 tablespoon olive oil
15 g (½ oz) butter
1 teaspoon crushed coriander seeds
4 spring onions, thinly sliced
400 g (13 oz) freshly cooked beetroot, cut into 1 cm (½ inch) dice
500 g (1 lb) risotto rice
1.5 litres (2½ pints) hot vegetable stock
200 g (7 oz) cream cheese
4 tablespoons finely chopped dill
salt and pepper

To garnish (optional):
dill sprigs

1 Heat the oil and butter in a 25 cm (10 inch) heavy-based saucepan. Add the coriander seeds and spring onions and stir-fry briskly for 1 minute.

2 Add the beetroot and the rice. Cook, stirring, for 2–3 minutes to coat all the grains with oil and butter. Pour in the hot stock a ladleful at a time, stirring often until each ladleful is absorbed before adding the next. This should take about 20 minutes, by which time the rice should be tender but still firm to the bite.

3 Stir in the cream cheese and dill, and season to taste. Serve immediately, garnished with dill sprigs, if liked.

Mixed vegetable curry

alcohol free ✓ | citrus free ✕ | dairy free ✓ | gluten free ✕ | wheat free ✕

Serves 4 as a main dish or 6 as a side dish
Preparation time: 15 minutes
Cooking time: 20–25 minutes

Per serving
Energy 133 kcals/550 kJ | Protein 3 g | Carbohydrate 11 g | Fat 9 g
Fibre 4 g

2–3 tablespoons vegetable oil
1 small onion, chopped, or 2 teaspoons cumin seeds
500 g (1 lb) mixed vegetables, such as potatoes, carrots, swede,
  peas, French beans, cauliflower, cut into chunks or broken into
  florets (French beans can be left whole)
1 teaspoon chilli powder
2 teaspoons ground coriander
½ teaspoon ground turmeric
salt
2–3 tomatoes, skinned and chopped, or juice of 1 lemon
300 ml (½ pint) water (optional)
naan, chappatis or basmati rice, to serve

1 Heat the oil in a heavy-based saucepan. Add the onion and fry over a medium heat, stirring occasionally, until light brown. Alternatively, fry the cumin seeds until they pop. Add the mixed vegetables and stir in the chilli powder, ground coriander, turmeric and salt to taste. Fry for 2–3 minutes.

2 Add the chopped tomatoes or the lemon juice. Stir well and add only a little water if you prefer a dry vegetable curry. Cover and cook gently for 10–12 minutes, until dry. For a moister curry, stir in 300 ml (½ pint) water then cover and simmer for 5–6 minutes, until the vegetables are tender.

3 Serve as a main dish with naan, chappatis or rice, or on its own as a side dish.

Vegetable tagine

alcohol free ✓ | citrus free ✓ | dairy free ✓ | gluten free ✓ | wheat free ✓

Serves 4
Preparation time: 15 minutes
Cooking time: 45 minutes

Per serving
Energy 109 kcals/459 kJ | Protein 4 g | Carbohydrate 15 g | Fat 4 g
Fibre 8 g

1 tablespoon virgin olive oil
1 red onion, cut into wedges
2 garlic cloves, crushed
3 celery sticks, sliced
3 carrots, thinly sliced
2 teaspoons Harissa (see page 213)
625 g (1¼ lb) small aubergines, chopped
2 large well-flavoured tomatoes, chopped
250 ml (8 fl oz) water
125 g (4 oz) small okra, trimmed
salt
chopped coriander leaves, to garnish

1 Heat the oil in a saucepan. Add the onion, garlic, celery and carrots and cook until beginning to brown. Add the harissa and stir for 1 minute.

2 Add the aubergines, tomatoes and the water to the pan. Bring to the boil, then cover the pan and simmer gently for about 25 minutes.

3 Stir the okra into the pan, cover and cook for 15–20 minutes, until the okra is tender.

4 If necessary, uncover the pan towards the end of cooking so that the consistency of the sauce is quite thick. Add salt to taste. To serve garnish with chopped coriander.

Charred asparagus with lemon, basil and spaghetti

alcohol free ✓ | citrus free ✗ | dairy free ✗ | gluten free ✗ | wheat free ✗

Serves 4
Preparation time: 10 minutes
Cooking time: 15 minutes

Per serving
Energy 464 kcals/1959 kJ | Protein 18 g | Carbohydrate 73 g | Fat 13 g
Fibre 7 g

500 g (1 lb) thin asparagus, trimmed
3–4 tablespoons extra virgin olive oil
juice of 1 lemon
375 g (12 oz) dried spaghetti
2 garlic cloves, roughly chopped
¼–½ teaspoon dried chilli flakes
25 g (1 oz) basil leaves
25 g (1 oz) freshly grated Parmesan cheese, plus extra to serve
salt and pepper

1 Brush the asparagus with a little oil and griddle or grill them until charred and tender. Toss with a little more oil, half of the lemon juice and salt and pepper and set aside.

2 Cook the pasta in a large pan of lightly salted boiling water, according to the packet instructions, until just tender.

3 Just before the pasta is cooked, heat the remaining oil in a large frying pan and sauté the garlic with a little salt for 3–4 minutes, until softened but not browned. Add the chilli flakes and asparagus and heat through.

4 Drain the pasta, reserving 4 tablespoons of the cooking liquid, and add both to the pan with the basil, the remaining lemon juice, pepper and Parmesan. Serve immediately, with extra Parmesan, if liked.

Tagliatelle with rocket and cherry tomato sauce

alcohol free ✓ | citrus free ✓ | dairy free ✗ | gluten free ✗ | wheat free ✗

Serves 4
Preparation time: 10 minutes
Cooking time: 8–12 minutes

Per serving
Energy 540 kcals/2256 kJ | Protein 17 g | Carbohydrate 95 g | Fat 10 g
Fibre 3 g

500 g (1 lb) dried tagliatelle verde
3 tablespoons olive oil
2 garlic cloves, finely chopped
500 g (1 lb) very ripe cherry tomatoes, halved
1 tablespoon balsamic vinegar
175 g (6 oz) rocket
salt and pepper
Parmesan cheese shavings, to serve

1 Bring at least 2 litres (3½ pints) of water to the boil in a large saucepan. Add a pinch of salt. Cook the pasta for 8–12 minutes, or according to the packet instructions, until just tender.

2 Meanwhile, heat the oil in a frying pan, add the garlic and cook for 1 minute until golden. Add the tomatoes and cook for barely 1 minute. The tomatoes should only just heat through and start to disintegrate.

3 Sprinkle the tomatoes with the balsamic vinegar, allow it to evaporate, then toss in the rocket. Carefully stir to mix it with the tomatoes and heat through so that the rocket is just wilted. Season well with salt and pepper, then toss with the cooked pasta. Cover with Parmesan shavings and serve immediately.

Harissa

alcohol free ✓ | citrus free ✓ | dairy free ✓ | gluten free ✓ | wheat free ✓

Serves 4
Preparation time: 20 minutes
Cooking time: 40 minutes

Whole recipe
Energy 180 kcals/747 kJ | Protein 4 g | Carbohydrate 15 g | Fat 13 g
Fibre 3 g

2 red peppers, roasted and skinned (see page 136)
25 g (1 oz) fresh red chillies, chopped, seeds retained
1–2 garlic cloves, crushed
½ teaspoon coriander seeds, toasted
2 teaspoons caraway seeds
olive oil
salt

1 Put the red peppers, the chillies and their seeds, garlic, coriander
and caraway seeds and a pinch of salt into a food processor or
blender and process, adding enough oil to make a thick paste.

2 Pack the harissa into a small, clean, dry jar and pour a layer of oil
over the top. Cover with a tight-fitting lid and keep in the
refrigerator, until required.

Puddings and cakes

Summer pudding

alcohol free ✓ | citrus free ✓ | dairy free ✗ | gluten free ✗ | wheat free ✗

Serves 8
Preparation time: 30 minutes, plus soaking and chilling
Cooking time: 15 minutes

Per serving
Energy 116 kcals/494 kJ | Protein 4 g | Carbohydrate 25 g | Fat 1 g
Fibre 8 g

500 g (1 lb) mixed blackberries and blackcurrants
3 tablespoons clear honey
125 g (4 oz) raspberries
125 g (4 oz) strawberries
8 slices wholemeal bread, crusts removed
low-fat natural yogurt, to serve

To decorate:
redcurrants
mint sprigs

1 Put the blackberries, blackcurrants and honey into a heavy-based saucepan and cook gently for 10–15 minutes, stirring occasionally, until tender. Add the raspberries and strawberries and leave to cool. Strain the fruit through a nylon sieve, reserving the juice.

2 Cut 3 circles of bread to fit the base, middle and top of a 900 ml (1½ pint) pudding basin. Shape the remaining bread to fit around the sides of the bowl. Soak all the bread in the reserved fruit juice.

3 Line the bowl bottom with the smallest bread circle, then arrange the shaped bread around the sides. Pour in half of the fruit and top with the middle-sized bread circle. Cover with the remaining fruit and the largest circle. Fold over any bread protruding from the basin.

4 Cover with a saucer small enough to fit inside the basin, and put a 500 g (1 lb) weight on top. Leave in the refrigerator overnight. Turn on to a serving plate and pour over any remaining fruit juice. Serve with yogurt, and decorate with redcurrants and mint sprigs.

Peach granita

alcohol free ✕ | citrus free ✕ | dairy free ✓ | gluten free ✓ | wheat free ✓

Serves 4
Preparation time: 15 minutes, plus freezing
Cooking time: 6 minutes

Per serving
Energy 75 kcals/ 318 kJ | Protein 3 g | Carbohydrate 11 g | Fat 0 g
Fibre 2 g

375 g (12 oz) ripe peaches
150 ml (¼ pint) dry white wine
150 ml (¼ pint) orange juice
2 egg whites
redcurrants, to decorate (optional)

1 Remove the skin from the peaches. Halve the fruit, removing the stones, and chop the flesh roughly.

2 Put the peach flesh into a saucepan with the white wine and orange juice. Simmer gently for 5 minutes, then blend the peaches and the liquid in a food processor or blender until smooth. Leave to cool. Put the mixture into a shallow container. Freeze until the granita is slushy around the edges, then tip into a bowl and break up the ice crystals.

3 Whisk the egg whites until stiff but not dry. Fold lightly but thoroughly into the partly frozen granita. Return to the container and freeze for 2–3 hours, until firm. Serve decorated with redcurrants, if liked.

Fig and honey pots

alcohol free ✓ | citrus free ✓ | dairy free ✕ | gluten free ✓ | wheat free ✓

Serves 4
Preparation time: 10 minutes, plus chilling

Per serving
Energy 284 kcals/1193 kJ | Protein 10 g | Carbohydrate 30 g | Fat 6 g
Fibre 2 g

6 fresh figs, thinly sliced
450 ml (¾ pint) Greek yogurt
4 tablespoons clear honey
2 tablespoons chopped pistachio nuts
2 fresh figs, cut into wedges, to decorate (optional)

1 Arrange the fig slices snugly in the bottom of 4 glasses or glass
bowls. Spoon the yogurt over the figs and chill for about
10–15 minutes.

2 Just before serving, drizzle 1 tablespoon of the honey over each
dessert and sprinkle chopped pistachio nuts on top. Decorate
with wedges of fig, if using.

Wholemeal pear tart

alcohol free ✓ I citrus free ✓ I dairy free ✗ I gluten free ✗ I wheat free ✗

Serves 6
Preparation time: 30 minutes, plus chilling
Cooking time: 40–50 minutes

Per serving

Energy 319 kcals/1340 kJ I Protein 5 g I Carbohydrate 46 g I Fat 14 g
Fibre 3 g

1 tablespoon clear honey, warmed, to glaze
redcurrants, to decorate

Pastry:
100 g (3½ oz) plain flour, sifted
100 g (3½ oz) wholemeal flour
100 g (3½ oz) sunflower margarine
2–2½ tablespoons cold water

Filling:
2 tablespoons raspberry jam (optional)
2 teaspoons custard powder
½–1 tablespoon caster sugar
150 ml (¼ pint) skimmed milk
425 g (14 oz) canned pear halves in natural juice, drained

1 To make the pastry, place the flours in a mixing bowl. Rub in the margarine until the mixture resembles fine breadcrumbs. Add the water, mix to make a firm dough and knead until smooth. Roll out two-thirds of the dough to make a circle large enough to line an 18 cm (7 inch) greased flan ring, then trim the edges. Put into the refrigerator for 10–15 minutes to chill.

2 Prick the base of the pastry case with a fork and bake blind in a preheated oven at 200°C (400°F), Gas Mark 6, for 10 minutes. Leave to cool, then spread the jam, if using, over the pastry base.

3 To make the custard, blend the powder and sugar with 1 tablespoon of the milk in a small bowl. Bring the rest of the milk to a boil in a small saucepan and pour it over the custard, stirring until thickened and smooth. Pour the custard into the flan ring and allow to set slightly. Arrange the pear halves around the edge of the pastry, rounded sides up.

4 Roll out the remaining dough to fit the flan ring. Dampen the edge of the pastry base. Put the pastry top on to the flan ring and press gently to seal the edges. Trim and flute the edges. Bake in the oven for 30–40 minutes.

5 Remove the flan ring and brush the tart with the warmed honey. Serve decorated with redcurrants.

Date and walnut bread

alcohol free ✓ | citrus free ✓ | dairy free ✕ | gluten free ✕ | wheat free ✕

Makes 1 x 500 g (1 lb) loaf
Preparation time: 15 minutes, plus standing
Cooking time: 55 minutes–1 hour

8 slices, per serving
Energy 218 kcals/920 kJ | Protein 7 g | Carbohydrate 37 g | Fat 6 g
Fibre 8 g

125 g (4 oz) breakfast bran
75 g (3 oz) molasses sugar
125 g (4 oz) dates, chopped
50 g (2 oz) walnuts, chopped
300 ml (½ pint) milk
125 g (4 oz) wholemeal flour
2 teaspoons baking powder

1 Put the breakfast bran, sugar, dates, walnuts, reserving some dates and walnuts for decoration, and milk into a mixing bowl. Stir well and leave for 1 hour. Add the flour, sift in the baking powder and mix together thoroughly.

2 Scoop the mixture into a lined and greased 500 g (1 lb) loaf tin and sprinkle over the reserved dates and walnuts. Bake in a preheated oven at 180°C (350°F), Gas Mark 4, for 55 minutes– 1 hour, until a skewer inserted into the centre comes out clean. Tip out the loaf to cool.

Fruit and nut crumble

alcohol free ✓ | citrus free ✓ | dairy free ✗ | gluten free ✗ | wheat free ✗

Serves 6
Preparation time: 15 minutes, plus soaking
Cooking time: 35–50 minutes

Per serving
Energy 394 kcals/1663 kJ | Protein 6 g | Carbohydrate 67 g | Fat 13 g
Fibre 15 g

175 g (6 oz) dried apricots
125 g (4 oz) dried pitted prunes
125 g (4 oz) dried figs
50 g (2 oz) dried apples
600 ml (1 pint) apple juice
100 g (3½ oz) wholemeal flour
50 g (2 oz) margarine
50 g (2 oz) muscovado or soft brown sugar, sifted
50 g (2 oz) hazelnuts, chopped
low-fat natural yogurt, to serve (optional)
rosemary sprigs, to garnish

1 Put the dried fruits into a bowl with the juice and leave overnight to soak. Simmer in a saucepan for 10–15 minutes, until softened. Turn into an ovenproof dish.

2 Sift the flour into a bowl and rub in the margarine until the mixture resembles breadcrumbs. Stir in the sugar, reserving a little to serve, and the hazelnuts, then sprinkle the crumble over the fruit.

3 Bake in a preheated oven at 200°F (400°C), Gas Mark 6, for 25–30 minutes. Serve with low-fat yogurt, if liked, sprinkled with the reserved sugar and garnished with rosemary sprigs.

Glossary

VITAMIN B6 Essential for the manufacture of serotonin.

VITAMINS C, E AND BETA-CAROTENE (which is converted into vitamin A in the body) These help to control the unstable molecules, free radicals, which can attack body cells.

CORPUS LUTEUM After an egg is released from a follicle in the ovary at ovulation, the empty follicle turns into the corpus luteum. It then releases hormones to prepare the body for pregnancy in case fertilization occurs.

ENDOMETRIUM The lining of the womb which builds up ready to receive a fertilized egg. If fertilization does not occur, the endometrium is shed in the form of a period.

FOLLICLE A sac in the ovary containing an egg or ovum. Each follicle contains one egg, which matures there before being released at ovulation.

FOLLICULAR PHASE Days six to fourteen of the menstrual cycle, when an egg develops in the ovary and is eventually released. During this phase, the endometrium also starts to grow and thicken.

FREE RADICALS Chemicals produced in the body which limit the effectiveness of the immune system. They are produced in response to atmospheric pollution and food additives, among many other things.

FSH Follicle stimulating hormone. It is released by the pituitary gland and causes the follicles in the ovaries to mature and produce a ripe egg.

HORMONES Chemical messengers that travel around in the bloodstream to act on cells and tissues around the body and tell them what to do. Each hormone is responsible for acting on one specific type of tissue only.

HYPOTHALAMUS Part of the base of the brain which controls many automatic body functions. It controls the menstrual cycle by releasing hormones into the blood.

LH Luteinizing hormone. A hormone produced by the pituitary gland, which causes one of the follicles in an ovary to release a ripe egg (ovulation).

LUTEAL PHASE Days 15–28 of the menstrual cycle, when PMS symptoms develop. The lining of the uterus becomes very thick and, if fertilization does not occur, it is sloughed off during menstruation.

MENSTRUAL CYCLE The time span from the first day of one menstrual period to the first day of the next one. It is usually between 24 and 40 days.

MENSTRUAL MAGNIFICATION The worsening of long-term medical conditions or mental health problems during the second half of the menstrual cycle.

MENSTRUAL PHASE Days one to five of the menstrual cycle when the lining of the womb is shed.

OESTROGEN One of the female sex hormones, which is produced by the ovaries and helps to regulate the menstrual cycle and reproductive function.

OVARIES Organs of the reproductive system, which produce and store eggs. The ovaries also produce the female sex hormones oestrogen and progesterone which regulate the menstrual cycle.

OVULATION The release of a ripe egg from an ovary.

PDD Premenstrual dysphoric disorder. A condition similar to PMS, except the symptoms are primarily related to mood. There are conflicting opinions among doctors on whether

PDD is a severe form of PMS, or a separate mood disorder tied to the menstrual cycle.

PITUITARY GLAND A gland in the brain which works with the hypothalamus to regulate the menstrual cycle.

PMS Premenstrual syndrome. The physical and emotional symptoms which many women experience in the second half of the menstrual cycle, just before their period.

PROGESTERONE One of the female sex hormones which, with oestrogen, regulates the menstrual cycle and paves the way for pregnancy.

PROGESTOGEN A synthetic form of progesterone, found in contraceptive pills and HRT.

SEROTONIN A brain chemical which helps to control mood. Low serotonin levels are linked to cravings for starchy foods, sleep disorders, depression and mood swings – all symptoms of PMS.

SSRIs Selective serotonin reuptake inhibitors, drugs which act to raise serotonin levels. The best-known is fluoxetine.

TRIGGER FACTOR Anything which triggers symptoms of PMS. Certain foods, stress, or coming off the pill, for example, can all be trigger factors of PMS.

UTERUS The womb.

General index

Recipe index